FITNESS FIRST
A 14-Day Diet & Exercise Program

FITNESS FIRST
A 14-Day Diet & Exercise Program

by
Jeanne Jones & Karma Kientzler

Medical Preface by Clifford W. Colwell, M.D.
Dietitian's Preface by Marilyn Majchrzak, M.S., R.D.
Drawings by Joe D'Addetta

101 Productions/San Francisco

Back Cover Photograph: Tim Fuller

Printed and bound in the United States of America. Distributed
to the book trade in the United States by Charles Scribner's
Sons, New York.

Published by 101 Productions
834 Mission Street
San Francisco, California 94103

Library of Congress Cataloging in Publication Data
Jones, Jeanne
  Fitness first.

  Bibliography: p.
  Includes index.
  1. Low-calorie diet—Recipes.   2. Reducing
exercises.   I. Kientzler, Karma, joint author.
II. Title.
RM222.2.J62   613.2'5   80-11320
ISBN 0-89286-167-3

TO ENID AND MEL ZUCKERMAN
for creating the opportunity for us to work together

In Grateful Acknowledgment:
Lee Ann Jones for recipe preparation and testing
Taita Pearn, M.S., R.D. for technical advice and professional assistance
Viola Stroup for technical and editorial assistance

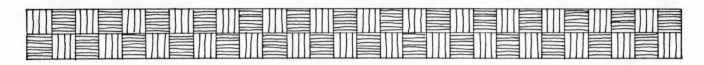

Contents

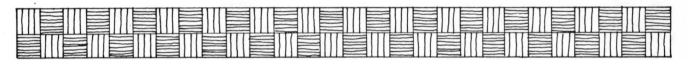

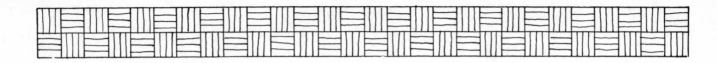

Medical Preface

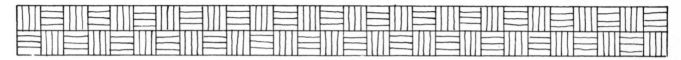

In the past decade, our health care delivery system has begun to recognize the importance of preventive medicine. Fundamental to this concept is a change in everyday behavior to promote your own health. Unfortunately, incorporating this idea into one's own daily life is difficult to accomplish. The goal is proper weight control and body fitness—the difficulty is in establishing an acceptable pathway. I believe that certain basic questions must be asked of any potential program.

• Is the overall philosophy compatible with your own, so that the program will be fun and interesting for you?
• Does the diet present a realistic method of reducing, and more importantly, of maintaining your weight with a well-balanced diet?
• Does the diet avoid the risks of pills or toxic substances which are likely to adversely affect your general health?
• Is the fitness program designed for "real" people with minimal time available to exercise each day?
• Does the exercise program promote total body fitness, and allow for progression as the individual increases his strength and endurance?

I personally applaud the *Fitness First* approach to dieting and exercise presented by Jeanne Jones and Karma Kientzler, and highly recommend this volume to the person who is serious about health achievement and maintenance. It is a commonsense, total fitness program with realistic guidelines and schedules, presented in an interesting and readable way. The goals outlined for a permanent "new you" are exciting and are achievable by all of us.

——Clifford W. Colwell, Jr., M.D.
Head, Division of Orthopedic Surgery
Scripps Clinic and Research Foundation
La Jolla, California

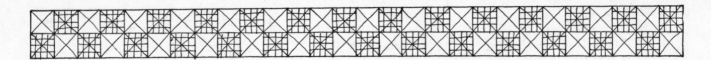

Dietitian's Preface

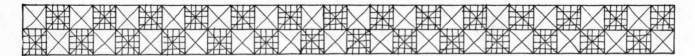

Searching a store for a book that presents a well-balanced weight reduction program can be a frustrating experience. As a nutritionist, I am constantly dismayed by the enormous amount of misinformation being passed on to the consumer.

Having read Jeanne Jones' previous books, which successfully address major health concerns facing the American public, I was excited and pleased to review this manuscript. This latest book offers sensible calorie restriction and exercise patterns, *plus* valuable information on some of the public's common health concerns—the presence of sodium, saturated fat and fiber in the diet.

Fitness First is a healthy approach to weight loss. The calorie restriction is sensible in relation to the percentage of fat, carbohydrate and protein provided. In view of the lowered calorie intake during the first 14 days, however, a multivitamin mineral supplement is recommended for keeping adequate nutrition standards and for health maintenance. It is also important that you have your doctor check your physical condition before you begin this program, and then follow the program precisely as described.

By following the *Fitness First* program you will not only achieve the immediate rewards of sensible weight loss and a trimmer body, but you will also develop sound nutrition habits and exercise patterns for a healthy lifetime.

——Marilyn Majchrzak, M.S., R.D.

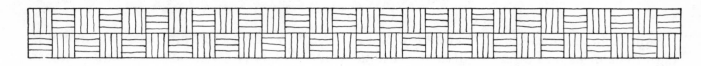

Introduction

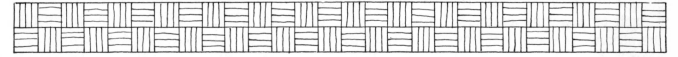

Fitness First is a dynamic approach to becoming the *you* that you have always wanted to be. In just 14 days you are going to look better, feel better, have more energy and more enthusiasm for life than ever before.

But this isn't where it stops. The truly sensational part of this program is that it can keep you looking and feeling better for the rest of your life. There is no way to take off unwanted pounds and inches overnight any more than it was possible for you to add those excess pounds and inches overnight. We believe that the *Fitness First* program is the fastest and most painless way to achieve a fit, trim body—a *permanent* new you.

The first week of the *Fitness First* diet is the brown-bag approach. No involved preparation is required and, except for Day One, the foods can be carried in a brown bag and the drinks in a jar or Thermos. The second week takes a more gourmet approach to weight reduction and recipes are given for all the suggested dishes. The menus and recipes for this week are designed as guidelines for people who want to serve their friends and families interesting and delicious meals without going off their diet programs. Additional low-calorie recipes are included in the recipe section to help in menu planning when you reach the *Fitness Forever* program.

The nutritional content and calories in the second week's menus are identical to those of the corresponding days of the first week, with the addition of one fat portion (see page 14) per day. Therefore, when you do not have time to prepare the suggested dishes in the second week, refer back to the same day in the first week for a less time-consuming approach to the meal. Conversely, during the first week if you wish to entertain your friends with a more elaborate approach to your diet, go to the same day of the second week and use that day's menu for your meal.

The recommended two quarts of water throughout the day are extremely important to remove any toxins present due to the weight reduction process. You will also find when drinking an adequate amount of water that your skin will improve markedly after just one week. The habit of added water consumption is one that should remain with you forever.

Alcoholic beverages are not allowed in the *Fitness First* diet program because alcohol is high in calories and offers so little nutritional value. The only other beverages allowed are tea and regular or decaffeinated coffee without cream or sugar, soda water or mineral water (see Counterfeit Cocktail, page 90). The caffeine in coffee and tea, however, tends to lower the blood sugar and will cause the feeling of hunger between meals. Herb teas are more highly recommended as a hot beverage. Diet sodas are not recommended because they are chemically laced products that offer no nutritional value and are in no way a natural approach to lowering calories. Between meals, or to add desired quantity to the meals themselves, you may eat any of the free foods indicated on the Vegetable Portion List on page 3.

It is important to follow this program exactly for the first 14 days. After reaching your initial goals in both weight and measurements and starting the *Fitness Forever* program, you may substitute the Day One liquid diet of either week when you feel you have overindulged.

At this point you may be asking yourself "What is the difference between the *Fitness First* diet program and all other reducing diets I have either read about or actually used?" The answer is that it is totally without gimmicks. There is no secret formula or magic combination of foods. It is a straightforward, commonsense approach to a perfectly balanced diet and exercise program within the capabilities of everyone considering time, money and ease. Plus, the usual grouchiness associated with weight-loss diets doesn't have to happen. But the best aspect of the *Fitness First* program is that you are going to remain happy for the rest of your life.

In just 14 days you will have acquired an understanding of menu planning and exercise that will bring you the realization of how much happier you are with your full commitment to *Fitness First*. There is no special equipment needed. There are no pills to be taken. The only suggestion aside from what is included here or for any other diet program is to check with your physician before beginning.

The very fact that you have taken the time to read this introduction shows that you are interested enough in your own self-improvement to try the *Fitness First* program. After 14 days we can almost promise you it will become not just *Fitness First*—but *Fitness Forever*.

——Jeanne Jones and Karma Kientzler

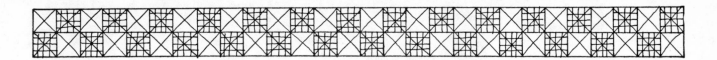

Diet Program

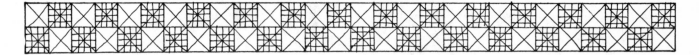

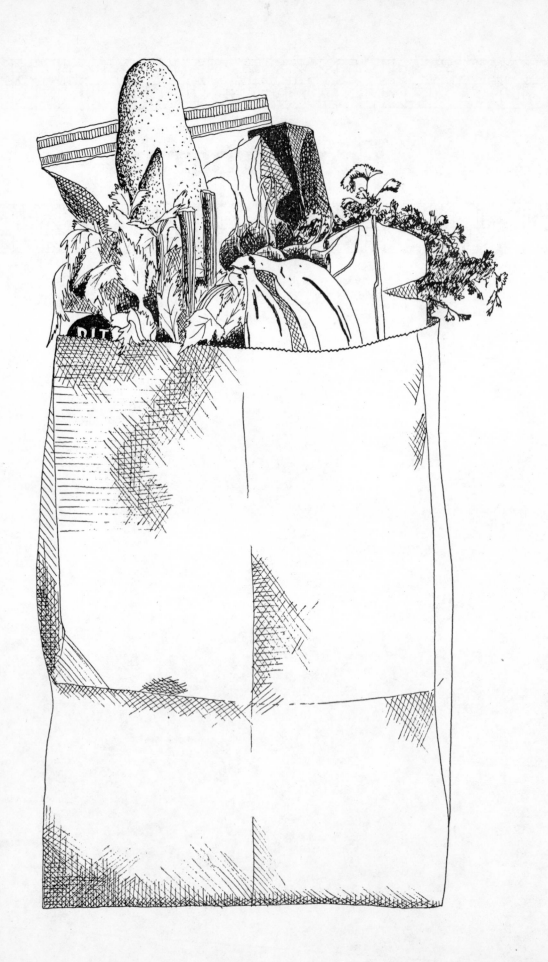

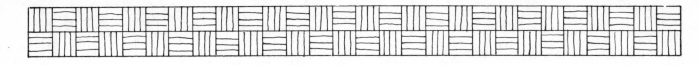

Food Portions

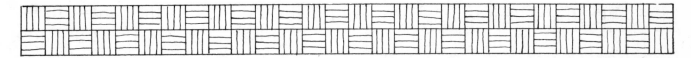

The food portion data that appears with each recipe is based on the exchange diet of the American Diabetes Association. In the exchange diet, numbers are rounded to the nearest whole digits to make it easier for laypersons to compute their calorie intake. For this reason, mathematical purists might be bothered by the fact that in most instances the percentages of the calories in the carbohydrate, protein and fat content will not total exactly 100 percent of the calories for the food group being calculated. The most important thing to remember is that a gram of fat is equal to 9 calories while a gram of either carbohydrate or protein is equal to 4 calories. It becomes easy to see why fat will indeed make you fat faster!

Drinking alcoholic beverages is discouraged in low-calorie diets because alcohol contains 7 calories per gram and contributes nothing nutritionally; therefore you are wasting precious calories needed for nutritionally beneficial foods.

ONE PORTION*	CALORIES	CARBOHYDRATE		PROTEIN		FAT	
		Grams	×4 Calories	Grams	×4 Calories	Grams	×9 Calories
Fruit	40	10	40 (100%)				
Vegetable	25	5	20 (80%)	2	4 (16%)		
Starch	70	15	60 (86%)	2	8 (12%)		
Low-fat Protein	55			7	28 (51%)	3	27 (49%)
Medium-fat Protein	75			7	28 (37%)	5	45 (60%)
High-fat Protein	95			7	28 (29%)	7	63 (66%)
Fat	45					5	45 (100%)
Non-fat Milk	80	12	48 (60%)	8	32 (40%)	Tr.	
Low-fat Milk	125	12	48 (38%)	8	32 (27%)	5	45 (36%)
Whole Milk	170	12	48 (28%)	8	32 (19%)	10	90 (53%)

*See following lists for portion sizes.

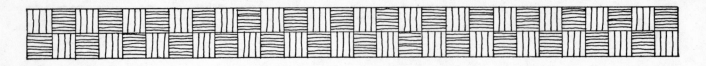

gm. fiber	mg. chol.	mg. sodium
= grams fiber	= milligrams cholesterol	= milligrams sodium

Fruit Portion List

Each portion below equals 1 Fruit Portion and contains approximately:

- 10 grams of carbohydrate
- 40 calories

   * good source of Vitamin C
  ** good source of Vitamin A
 *** good source of Vitamins A and C
 †† figures not available

gm. fiber	mg. chol.	mg. sodium	
1.0	0	1	Apple: 1 2 inches in diameter
.1	0	.7	Apple juice: 1/3 cup
.6	0	2	Applesauce, unsweetened: 1/2 cup
.6	0	1	Apricots, fresh: 2 medium**
.5	0	3	Apricots, dried: 3 halves**
			Avocado: see Fat Portion List
.3	0	.5	Banana: 1/2 small
2.0	0	1	Blackberries: 1/2 cup
1.1	0	1	Blueberries: 1/2 cup
.3	0	10	Cantaloupe: 1/4 6 inches in diameter***
.3	0	1	Cherries, sweet: 10 large
††	0	2	Cranberries, unsweetened: 1 cup
.3	0	††	Crenshaw melon: 2-inch wedge
.5	0	2	Dates: 2
.5	0	2	Date "sugar": 1 tablespoon
.6	0	1	Figs, fresh: 1 large
.8	0	7	Figs, dried: 1 large
0	0	0	Fructose: 1 tablespoon
.2	0	1	Grapefruit: 1/2 4 inches in diameter*
Tr.	0	1	Grapefruit juice: 1/2 cup*
.4	0	2	Grapes: 12 large
.2	0	2	Grapes, Thompson Seedless: 20 grapes

gm. fiber	mg. chol.	mg. sodium	
Tr.	0	1	Grape juice: 1/4 cup
4.4	0	2	Guava: 2/3*
0	0	1	Honey: 2 teaspoons
.7	0	27	Honeydew melon: 1/4 5 inches in diameter
.4	0	††	Kiwi: 1 medium
3.0	0	6	Kumquats: 2
Tr.	0	1	Lemon juice: 1/2 cup
Tr.	0	1	Lime juice: 1/2 cup
.5	0	††	Loquats: 3
.2	0	3	Litchi nuts, fresh: 3
.9	0	3	Mango: 1/2 small**
††	0	18	Molasses, blackstrap: 1 tablespoon
.3	0	8	Nectarine: 1 medium
.5	0	1	Orange: 1 small*
.1	0	1	Orange juice: 1/2 cup*
1.0	0	3	Papaya: 1/3 medium*
1.5	0	16	Passionfruit: 1
.1	0	††	Passionfruit juice: 1/3 cup
.6	0	1	Peach: 1 medium
1.0	0	3	Pear: 1 small
.8	0	3	Persimmon: 1/2 medium
.3	0	1	Pineapple, fresh or canned without sugar: 1/2 cup
Tr.	0	1	Pineapple juice: 1/3 cup
.2	0	6	Plantain: 1/2 small
.3	0	2	Plums: 2 medium
.2	0	3	Pomegranate: 1 small
.3	0	2	Prunes, fresh or dried: 2
Tr.	0	5	Prune juice: 1/4 cup
.2	0	6	Raisins: 2 tablespoons
3.0	0	1	Raspberries: 1/2 cup
1.5	0	1	Strawberries: 3/4 cup
0	0	0	Sucrose: 1 tablespoon
.5	0	2	Tangerines: 1 large or 2 small
.5	0	1.5	Watermelon: 3/4 cup

Vegetable Portion List

Each portion below equals 1 Vegetable Portion, is equal to 1 cup unless otherwise specified, and contains approximately:

- 5 grams of carbohydrate
- 2 grams of protein
- 25 calories

* good source of Vitamin C
** good source of Vitamin A
*** good source of Vitamins A and C
† calories negligible when eaten raw
†† figures not available

gm. fiber	mg. chol.	mg. sodium	
.6	0	††	Alfalfa sprouts†
4.8	0	40	Artichoke, whole, base and ends of leaves (1 small)
1.0	0	1	Asparagus†
.7	0	4	Bean sprouts†
.8	0	40	Beets (1/2 cup)
1.3	0	37	Beet greens
††	0	8	Breadfruit (1/4 cup)
1.5	0	22	Broccoli***†
1.6	0	16	Brussels sprouts*
.8	0	16	Cabbage*†
1.0	0	24	Carrots (medium), 1**
1.0	0	12	Cauliflower†
.6	0	100	Celery†
.7	0	100	Celery root (1/2 cup)
.9	0	166	Chard†
.8	0	12	Chayote
.9	0	††	Chicory**†
2.0	0	42	Chilies†
1.2	0	16	Chives***†
.9	0	56	Collard*†
1.4	0	††	Coriander (Cilantro)†
.6	0	8	Cucumber†
1.6	0	80	Dandelion greens†
1.8	8	2	Eggplant
1.2	0	10	Endive†
1.0	0	10	Escarole**†
††	0	10	Garlic (1/4 cup)
.5	0	3	Green beans: see String beans
1.0	0	8	Green onion tops†
.5	0	††	Jerusalem artichokes (1/2 cup)
††	0	††	Jicama
1.2	0	48	Kale*†
.7	0	12	Leeks (1/2 cup)
.6	0	7	Lettuce†
1.8	0	.5	Lima beans, baby (1/4 cup)
††	0	††	Mint†
.8	0	10	Mushrooms†
.9	0	12	Mustard, fresh*†
1.0	0	4	Okra
.6	0	9	Onions (1/2 cup)
1.2	0	††	Palm heart
1.5	0	32	Parsley***†
.75	0	.4	Peas (1/4 cup)
††	0	Tr.	Pea pods (1/2 cup)
1.5	0	20	Peppers, green and red*†
††	0	8	Pimiento (1/2 cup)
.9	0	††	Poke†
1.3	0	2	Pumpkin (1/2 cup)*
.7	0	20	Radishes†
.9	0	2	Rhubarb†
.7	0	4	Romaine lettuce†
1.1	0	4	Rutabagas (1/2 cup)
††	0	9	Shallots (1/2 cup)
.9	0	37	Spinach†
1.2	0	1	Squash, acorn (1/2 cup)
1.2	0	1	Squash, Hubbard (1/2 cup)
††	0	2	Squash, spaghetti
1.2	0	6	String beans
1.2	0	2	Summer squash†
.9	0	6	Tomatoes (1 medium)
††	0	15	Tomatoes, canned in juice, unsalted (1/2 cup)
.1	0	282	Tomato catsup, regular (1 1/2 tablespoons)
††	0	6	Tomato catsup, dietetic, low-sodium (1 1/2 tablespoons)
.4	0	244	Tomato juice (1/2 cup)
††	0	26	Tomato juice, unsalted (1/2 cup)
.3	0	186	Tomato paste (2 tablespoons)
††	0	12	Tomato paste, unsalted (3 tablespoons)
.6	0	831	Tomato sauce (1/2 cup)
††	0	42	Tomato sauce, unsalted (1/2 cup)
.8	0	27	Turnips (1/2 cup)
.3	0	550	V-8 juice (2/3 cup)**
††	0	49	V-8 juice, unsalted (2/3 cup)**
.2	0	8	Water chestnuts (medium) (4)
.7	0	16	Watercress**†
1.4	0	1	Zucchini squash†

Starch Portion List

Each portion below equals 1 Starch Portion and contains approximately:

  15 grams of carbohydrate
  2 grams of protein
  70 calories

** good source of Vitamin A
†† figures not available

Vegetables

gm. fiber	mg. chol.	mg. sodium	
1.4	0	3	Beans, dried, cooked, unsalted (lima, soya, navy, pinto, kidney): 1/2 cup
.5	0	1.5	Beans, baked, without salt or pork: 1/4 cup
.6	0	1	Corn, on-the-cob: 1 4 inches long
.6	0	1	Corn, cooked and drained: 1/3 cup
.1	0	††	Hominy: 1/2 cup
.7	0	14	Lentils, dried, cooked: 1/2 cup
2.0	0	8	Parsnips: 1 small
.5	0	13	Peas, dried, cooked (black-eyed, split): 1/2 cup
.7	0	7	Potatoes, sweet, yams: 1/4 cup**
.5	0	2	Potatoes, white, baked or boiled: 1 2 inches in diameter
.5	0	2	Potatoes, white, mashed: 1/2 cup
.2	0	300	Potato chips: 15 2 inches in diameter
2.6	0	4	Pumpkin, canned: 1 cup
.2	0	6	Rice, brown, cooked, unsalted: 1/3 cup
Tr.	0	3	Rice, white, cooked, unsalted: 1/2 cup
††	0	4	Rice, wild, cooked, unsalted: 1/2 cup
.2	0	564	Tomato catsup, commercial: 3 tablespoons
††	0	12	Tomato catsup, dietetic, low sodium, 3 tablespoons

Breads

gm. fiber	mg. chol.	mg. sodium	
Tr.	0	††	Bagel: 1/2
Tr.	0	185	Biscuit: 1 2 inches in diameter
††	0	7	Bread, low sodium: 1 slice
.1	0	139	Bread, rye: 1 slice
.4	0	136	Bread, whole wheat: 1 slice
Tr.	0	148	Bread (white and sourdough): 1 slice
Tr.	0	200	Breadsticks: 4 7 inches long
Tr.	0	116	Bun, hamburger: 1/2
Tr.	0	153	Bun, hot dog: 2/3
.1	0	245	Corn bread: 1 piece 1 1/2 inches square
.3	0	††	Cracked wheat (bulgur): 1 1/2 tablespoons
Tr.	0	140	Croutons, plain: 1/2 cup
††	0	7	Croutons, plain, low-sodium bread: 1/2 cup
Tr.	0	133	English muffin: 1/2
Tr.	0	1	Matzo cracker, plain: 1 6 inches in diameter
Tr.	0	222	Melba toast: 6 slices
Tr.	0	117	Muffin, unsweetened: 1 2 inches in diameter
Tr.	0	412	Pancakes: 2 3 inches in diameter
††	0	7	Pancakes, low sodium: 2 3 inches in diameter
Tr.	0	88	Popover: 1
Tr.	0	143	Roll: 1 2 inches in diameter
Tr.	0	70	Rusks: 2
.1	0	712	Spoon bread: 1/2 cup
.3	0	Tr.	Tortilla, corn, flour: 1 7 inches in diameter
Tr.	0	203	Waffle: 1 4 inches in diameter

Cereals

gm. fiber	mg. chol.	mg. sodium	
2.4	0	287	All-Bran: 1/2 cup
2.0	0	94	Bran Flakes: 1/2 cup
3.3	0	††	Bran, unprocessed rice: 1/3 cup
3.2	0	††	Bran, unprocessed wheat: 1/3 cup
.2	0	240	Cheerios: 1 cup
.2	0	††	Concentrate: 1/4 cup
.1	0	178	Corn Flakes: 2/3 cup
.1	0	1	Cornmeal, cooked: 1/2 cup
Tr.	0	1	Cream-of-Wheat, cooked: 1/2 cup
.4	0	147	Grapenuts: 1/4 cup
.3	0	113	Grapenut Flakes: 1/2 cup
.1	0	1	Grits, cooked: 1/2 cup
Tr.	0	165	Kix: 3/4 cup
.3	0	132	Life: 1/2 cup
Tr.	0	1	Malt-O-Meal, cooked: 1/2 cup
Tr.	0	2	Maypo, cooked: 1/2 cup
Tr.	0	1	Matzo meal, cooked: 1/2 cup
.2	0	1	Oatmeal, cooked: 1/2 cup
.2	0	92	Pep: 1/2 cup
.2	0	1	Puffed rice: 1 1/2 cups

gm. fiber	mg. chol.	mg. sodium	
.3	0	1	Puffed wheat: 1½ cups
Tr.	0	174	Rice Krispies: ⅔ cup
.4	0	1	Shredded wheat, biscuit: 1 large
.3	0	168	Special K: 1¼ cups
.2	0	1	Steel cut oats, cooked: ½ cup
.4	0	163	Wheat Chex: ½ cup
Tr.	0	1	Wheat germ, defatted: 1 ounce or 3 tablespoons
.2	0	210	Wheaties: ⅔ cup

Flours

gm. fiber	mg. chol.	mg. sodium	
Tr.	0	2	Arrowroot: 2 tablespoons
Tr.	0	1	All purpose: 2½ tablespoons
Tr.	0	138	Bisquick: 1½ tablespoons
3.2	0	††	Bran, unprocessed wheat: 5 tablespoons
.3	0	1	Buckwheat: 3 tablespoons
Tr.	0	1	Cake: 2½ tablespoons
.1	0	Tr.	Cornmeal: 3 tablespoons
Tr.	0	Tr.	Cornstarch: 2 tablespoons
Tr.	0	1	Matzo meal: 3 tablespoons
Tr.	0	12	Potato flour: 2½ tablespoons
.5	0	1	Rye, dark: 4 tablespoons
.6	0	1	Whole wheat: 3 tablespoons
Tr.	0	1	Noodles, macaroni, spaghetti, cooked: ½ cup
Tr.	9.4	2	Noodles, dry, egg: 3½ ounces
Tr.	3.1	1.5	Noodles, cooked, egg: 3½ ounces

Crackers

gm. fiber	mg. chol.	mg. sodium	
Tr.	0	††	Animal: 8
Tr.	0	33	Arrowroot: 3
Tr.	0	††	Cheese tidbits: ½ cup
.2	0	88	Graham: 2
††	0	10	Low sodium: 4
Tr.	0	220	Oyster: 20 or ½ cup
Tr.	0	90	Pretzels: 10 very thin, or 1 large
Tr.	0	250	Saltines: 5, salted
Tr.	0	69	Soda: 3, unsalted
Tr.	0	192	Ritz: 6
.3	0	225	RyKrisp: 3
.3	0	130	Rye thins: 10
Tr.	0	336	Triangle thins: 14
††	0	150	Triscuits: 5
Tr.	0	††	Vegetable thins: 12
Tr.	0	276	Wheat thins: 12

Miscellaneous

gm. fiber	mg. chol.	mg. sodium	
1.8	0	10	Cocoa, dry, unsweetened: 2½ tablespoons
††	0	120	Fritos: ¾ ounce or ½ cup
0	26.3	40	Ice cream, low saturated fat: ½ cup
.3	0	1	Popcorn, popped, unbuttered and unsalted: 1½ cups

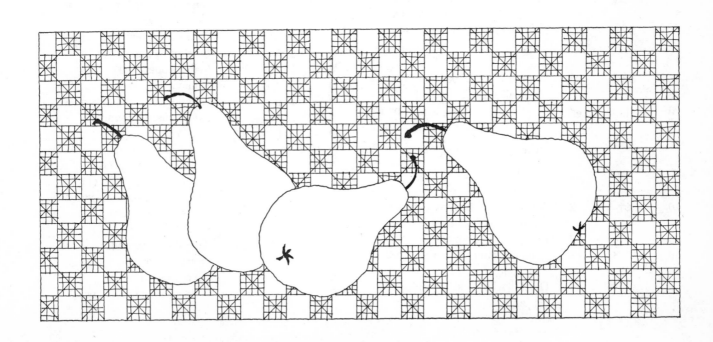

Low-fat Protein Portion List

Each portion below equals 1 Low-fat Protein Portion and contains approximately:

- 7 grams of protein
- 3 grams of fat
- 55 calories

†† figures not available

Cheese

gm. fiber	mg. chol.	mg. sodium	
0	2.6	234	Cottage cheese, low-fat: 1/4 cup
0	††	††	Cottage cheese, dry curd: 1/4 cup
0	††	222	Farmer's: 1/4 cup, crumbled, salted
0	3.0	75	Farmer's: 1/4 cup, crumbled, unsalted
0	3.0	††	Hoop: 1/4 cup
0	3.0	12	Pot: 1/4 cup
0	18.2	46	Ricotta, part skim: 1/4 cup or 2 ounces

Egg Substitutes

gm. fiber	mg. chol.	mg. sodium	
0	0	130	Liquid egg substitute: 1/4 cup (sodium content varies with brands)
0	0	††	Dry egg substitute: 3 tablespoons

Chicken

gm. fiber	mg. chol.	mg. sodium	
0	25.8	22	Broiled or roasted: 1 ounce or 1 slice 3×2×1/8 inch
0	22.4	19	Breast, without skin: 1/2 small, 1 ounce or 1/4 cup, chopped
0	25.8	25	Leg: 1/2 medium or 1 ounce

Turkey

gm. fiber	mg. chol.	mg. sodium	
0	22.4	23	Meat, white, without skin: 1 ounce or 1 slice 3×2×1/8 inch
0	††	28	Meat, dark, without skin: 1 ounce or 1 slice 3×2×1/8 inch

Other Poultry and Game

gm. fiber	mg. chol.	mg. sodium	
0	30.0	25	Buffalo: 1 ounce or 1 slice 3×2×1/8 inch
0	††	22	Cornish game hen, without skin: 1/4 bird or 1 ounce
0	††	20	Pheasant: 1 1/2 ounces
0	25.8	18	Rabbit: 1 ounce or 1 slice 3×2×1/8 inch
0	††	12	Quail, without skin: 1/4 bird or 1 ounce
0	††	22	Squab, without skin: 1/4 bird or 1 ounce
0	††	25	Venison, lean, roast or steak: 1 ounce or 1 slice 3×2×1/8 inch

Fish and Seafood

gm. fiber	mg. chol.	mg. sodium	
0	24.4	††	Abalone: 1 1/3 ounces
0	18.3	112	Albacore, canned in oil: 1 ounce
0	21.4	††	Anchovy fillets: 9
0	††	1540	Anchovy paste: 1 tablespoon
0	27.1	15	Bass: 1 1/2 ounces
0	85.7	624	Caviar: 1 ounce
0	††	††	Clam juice: 1 1/2 cups
0	18.0	51	Clams, fresh: 3 large or 1 1/2 ounces
0	27.0	††	Clams, canned: 1 1/2 ounces
0	18.1	31	Cod: 1 ounce
0	43.0	77	Crab, canned: 1/2 ounce
0	42.5	90	Crab, cracked, fresh: 1 1/2 ounces
0	30.2	110	Flounder: 1 2/3 ounces
0	55.0	††	Frog legs: 2 large or 3 ounces
0	18.1	30	Halibut: 1 ounce or 1 piece 2×2×1 inch
0	27.0	††	Herring, pickled: 1 1/4 ounces
0	††	2207	Herring, smoked: 1 1/4 ounces
0	31.0	90	Lobster, fresh: 1 1/2 ounces, 1/4 cup or 1/4 small lobster
0	36.0	90	Lobster, canned, unsalted: 1 1/2 ounces
0	23.0	31	Oysters, fresh: 3 medium or 1 1/2 ounces
0	25.5	171	Oysters, canned: 1 1/2 ounces
0	27.1	39	Perch: 1 1/2 ounces
0	27.1	38	Red snapper: 1 1/2 ounces
0	18.4	14	Salmon: 1 ounce
0	16.0	235	Salmon, canned: 1 1/2 ounces
0	24.4	33	Sand dabs: 1 1/2 ounces
0	40.0	108	Sardines: 4 small
0	††	26	Sardines, unsalted: 4 small
0	23.0	112	Scallops: 3 medium or 1 1/2 ounces
0	48.0	60	Shrimp, fresh: 5 medium
0	64.0	††	Shrimp, canned: 5 medium or 1 1/2 ounces
0	30.0	44	Sole: 1 2/3 ounces
0	27.1	††	Swordfish: 1 1/2 ounces
0	27.1	11	Trout: 1 1/2 ounces
0	18.1	10	Tuna, fresh: 1 ounce
0	††	370	Tuna, canned in oil: 1/4 cup

gm. fiber	mg. chol.	mg. sodium	
0	††	25	Tuna, unsalted, water packed (dietetic): 1/4 cup
0	27.1	32	Turbot: 1 1/2 ounces

Beef

gm. fiber	mg. chol.	mg. sodium	
0	41.8	26	Flank steak: 1 1/2 ounces
0	31.3	17	Rib roast: 1 ounce, 1/4 cup, chopped, or 1 slice $3 \times 2 \times 1/8$ inch
0	30.0	17	Steak, very lean (filet mignon, New York, sirloin, T-bone): 1 ounce or 1 slice $3 \times 2 \times 1/8$ inch
0	††	21	Tripe: 1 ounce or 1 piece 5×2 inches

Lamb

gm. fiber	mg. chol.	mg. sodium	
0	28.0	20	Chops, lean: 1/2 small chop or 1 ounce
0	27.7	20	Roast, lean: 1 ounce, 1 slice $3 \times 2 \times 1/8$ inch, or 1/4 cup, chopped

Pork

gm. fiber	mg. chol.	mg. sodium	
0	25.3	264	Ham: 1 ounce or 1 slice $3 \times 2 \times 1/8$ inch

Veal

gm. fiber	mg. chol.	mg. sodium	
0	28.7	23	Chop: 1/2 small or 1 ounce
0	29.0	23	Cutlet: 1 ounce or 1 slice $3 \times 2 \times 1/8$ inch
0	28.7	23	Roast: 1 ounce or 1 slice $3 \times 2 \times 1/8$ inch

---

Medium-fat Protein Portion List

Each portion below equals 1 Medium-fat Protein Portion and contains approximately:

    7 grams of protein
    5 grams of fat
    75 calories

Cheese

gm. fiber	mg. chol.	mg. sodium	
0	8.4	130	Cottage cheese, creamed: 1/4 cup
0	16.0	††	Feta: 1 ounce
0	17.4	227	Mozzarella: 1 ounce
0	14.8	163	Parmesan: 1/4 cup, 2/3 ounce or 4 tablespoons
0	29.1	46	Ricotta, regular: 1/4 cup or 2 ounces
0	14.8	247	Romano: 1/4 cup, 2/3 ounce or 4 tablespoons

Eggs

gm. fiber	mg. chol.	mg. sodium	
0	250.0	59	Eggs, medium: 1
0	0	47	Egg white: 1 (not a whole portion)
0	250.0	12	Egg yolk: 1 (not a whole portion)

Chicken

gm. fiber	mg. chol.	mg. sodium	
0	††	16	Gizzard: 1 ounce
0	††	20	Heart: 1 ounce
0	211.4	17	Liver: 1 ounce

Beef

gm. fiber	mg. chol.	mg. sodium	
0	571.4	54	Brains: 1 ounce
0	26.0	298	Corned beef, canned: 1 ounce or 1 slice $3 \times 2 \times 1/8$ inch
0	30.3	14	Hamburger, very lean (4 ounces raw=3 ounces cooked): 1 ounce
0	42.8	30	Heart: 1 ounce or 1 slice $3 \times 2 \times 1/8$ inch
0	107.1	72	Kidney: 1 ounce or 1 slice $3 \times 2 \times 1/8$ inch
0	124.1	59	Liver: 1 ounce or 1 slice $3 \times 2 \times 1/8$ inch
0	††	17	Tongue: 1 slice $3 \times 2 \times 1/4$ inch

Pork

gm. fiber	mg. chol.	mg. sodium	
0	25.3	343	Canadian bacon: 1 slice 2 1/2 inches in diameter, 1/4 inch thick
0	25.0	18	Chops, lean: 1/2 small chop or 1 ounce
0	††	19	Heart: 1 ounce
0	124.1	30	Liver: 1 ounce
0	25.0	18	Roast, lean: 1 ounce, 1 slice $3 \times 2 \times 1/8$ inch or 1/4 cup, chopped

Veal

gm. fiber	mg. chol.	mg. sodium	
0	124.1	30	Calves' liver: 1 ounce or 1 slice $3 \times 2 \times 1/8$ inch
0	71.4	33	Sweetbreads: 1 ounce, 1/4 pair or 1/4 cup, chopped
0	28.7	22	Roast, lean: 1 ounce, 1/4 cup, chopped, or 1 slice $3 \times 2 \times 1/8$ inch

High-fat Protein Portion List

Each portion below equals 1 High-fat Protein Portion and contains approximately:

    7 grams of protein
    7 grams of fat
    95 calories

†† figures not available

Cheese

gm. fiber	mg. chol.	mg. sodium	
0	28.4	193	American: 1 ounce
0	21.16	510	Bleu: 1 ounce or 1/4 cup, crumbled
0	30.1	193	Cheddar: 1 ounce
0	††	10	Cheddar, low sodium: 1 ounce (sodium content varies with brands)
0	29.1	204	Edam: 1 ounce
0	21.0	271	Liederkranz: 1 ounce
0	18.0	204	Monterey Jack: 1 ounce
0	25.0	204	Muenster: 1 ounce
Tr.	18.2	465	Pimiento cheese spread: 1 ounce
0	24.0	465	Roquefort: 1 ounce or 1/4 cup, crumbled
0	21.0	††	Stilton: 1 ounce or 1/4 cup, crumbled
0	28.0	85	Swiss: 1 ounce

Cold Cuts

gm. fiber	mg. chol.	mg. sodium	
0	25.9	266	Bologna: 1 ounce or 1 slice 4 1/2 inches in diameter, 1/8 inch thick
0	††	264	Liverwurst: 1 slice 3 inches in diameter, 1/4 inch thick
0	25.9	340	Spam: 1 ounce
0	25.9	425	Salami: 1 ounce or 1 slice 4 inches in diameter, 1/3 inch thick
0	25.9	228	Vienna sausage: 2 1/2 sausages or 1 ounce

Duck

gm. fiber	mg. chol.	mg. sodium	
0	††	21	Roasted, without skin: 1 ounce or 1 slice 3×2×1/8 inch
0	††	28	Wild duck, without skin: 1 ounce

Beef

gm. fiber	mg. chol.	mg. sodium	
0	31.3	17	Brisket: 1 ounce
0	25.9	508	Frankfurters: 1 (8 to 9 per pound)
0	31.3	18	Short ribs, very lean: 1 rib or 1 ounce

Peanut Butter

gm. fiber	mg. chol.	mg. sodium	
.3	0	156	Peanut butter, regular: 2 tablespoons
.3	0	6	Peanut butter, unsalted: 2 tablespoons

Pork

gm. fiber	mg. chol.	mg. sodium	
			Bacon: see Fat Portion List
0	25.9	250	Sausage, 2 small or 1 ounce
0	25.3	19	Spareribs, without fat: meat from 3 medium or 1 ounce

Fat Portion List

Each portion below equals 1 Fat Portion and contains approximately:

    5 grams of fat
    45 calories

†† figures not available

gm. fiber	mg. chol.	mg. sodium	
.8	0	1	Avocado: 1/8 4 inches in diameter
0	7.0	209	Bacon, crisp: 1 slice
0	12.0	39	Butter: 1 teaspoon
0	††	.3	Butter, unsalted: 1 teaspoon
1.2	††	5	Caraway seeds: 2 tablespoons
1.2	††	5	Cardamom seeds: 2 tablespoons
0	0	4	Chocolate, bitter: 1/3 ounce or 1/3 square
0	10.0	35	Cream cheese: 1 tablespoon
0	20.0	12	Cream, light, coffee: 2 tablespoons
0	20.0	5	Cream, heavy, whipping: 1 tablespoon
0	17.0	18	Cream, half-and-half: 3 tablespoons
0	16.0	12	Cream, sour: 2 tablespoons
0	0	32	Cream, sour, imitation: 2 tablespoons (Imo, Matey)
0	0	35	Margarine, polyunsaturated: 1 teaspoon
0	0	.8	Margarine, polyunsaturated, unsalted: 1 teaspoon
0	2.6	25	Mayonnaise: 1 teaspoon
0	0	0	Oils, polyunsaturated: 1 teaspoon
.6	††	125	Olives, ripe: 5 small
††	††	384	Olives, green: 4 medium
.8	††	3	Poppy seeds: 1 1/2 tablespoons

gm. fiber	mg. chol.	mg. sodium	
.2	††	††	Pumpkin seeds: 1½ teaspoons
			Salad dressings, commercial
.Tr.	††	59	Bleu cheese: 1 teaspoon
Tr.	††	95	Bleu cheese, diet, sugar free: 1 teaspoon
Tr.	††	57	Caesar: 1 teaspoon
Tr.	††	77	French: 1 teaspoon
Tr.	††	74	Italian: 1 teaspoon
Tr.	††	64	Italian, diet: 1 teaspoon
Tr.	††	48	Roquefort: 1 teaspoon
Tr.	††	44	Thousand island, diet: 1 teaspoon
Tr.	††	33	Thousand island, egg-free: 1 teaspoon
			Sauces, commercial
Tr.	††	††	Bearnaise: 1 teaspoon
Tr.	††	28	Hollandaise: 1 teaspoon
Tr.	††	61	Tartar: 1 teaspoon
.2	0	4	Sesame seeds: 2 teaspoons
.2	0	3	Sunflower seeds: 1½ teaspoons

Nuts, Unsalted

gm. fiber	mg. chol.	mg. sodium	
.3	0	.5	Almonds: 7
.2	0	.5	Brazil nuts: 2
.2	0	2	Cashews: 7
.5	0	5	Coconut, fresh: 1 piece 1×1× 3/8 inch
.3	0	5	Coconut, shredded, unsweetened: 2 tablespoons
1.2	0	.5	Filberts: 5
1.2	0	.5	Hazelnuts: 5
.1	0	††	Hickory nuts: 7 small
.3	0	††	Macadamia nuts: 2
.4	0	1	Peanuts, Spanish: 20
.4	0	1	Peanuts, Virginia: 10
.3	0	Tr.	Pecans: 6 halves
.2	0	††	Pine nuts: 1 tablespoon
.1	0	††	Pistachio nuts: 15
.2	0	††	Soy nuts, toasted: 3 tablespoons
.2	0	.5	Walnuts, black: 5 halves
.2	0	.5	Walnuts, California: 5 halves

Non-fat Milk Portion List

Each portion below equals 1 Non-fat Milk Portion and contains approximately:

12 grams of carbohydrate
8 grams of protein
trace of fat
80 calories

gm. fiber	mg. chol.	mg. sodium	
0	7.8	280	Buttermilk: 1 cup
0	††	155	Milk, powdered, skim, dry: 3 tablespoons
0	1.7	115	Milk, powdered, skim, mixed: 1/4 cup
0	††	6	Milk, powdered, low sodium (Featherweight): 3 tablespoons, dry, or 1 cup, mixed
0	2.3	127	Milk, skim, non-fat: 1 cup
0	††	121	Milk, skim, instant: 1 cup
0	2.3	165	Milk, evaporated, skim: 1/2 cup
0	††	75	Sherbet: 1 cup
0	††	116	Yogurt, plain, non-fat: 1 cup

Low-fat Milk Portion List

Each portion below equals 1 Low-fat Milk Portion and contains approximately:

12 grams of carbohydrate
8 grams of protein
5 grams of fat
125 calories

gm. fiber	mg. chol.	mg. sodium	
0	15.5	150	Milk, low-fat, 2% fat: 1 cup
0	††	12.5	Milk, Carnation Lo-Sodium Modified: 1 cup
0	17.0	115	Yogurt, plain, low-fat: 1 cup
0	††	141	Yogurt, flavored, low-fat: 1 cup

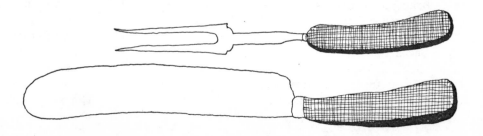

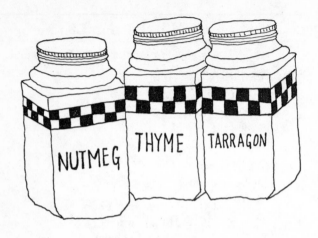

Whole Milk Portion List

Each portion below equals 1 Whole Milk Portion and contains approximately:

- 12 grams of carbohydrate
- 8 grams of protein
- 10 grams of fat
- 170 calories

gm. fiber	mg. chol.	mg. sodium	
0	26.0	136	Ice milk: 1 cup
0	32.7	120	Milk, whole: 1 cup
0	32.7	149	Milk, evaporated, whole: 1/2 cup
0	††	6	Milk, low-sodium Lonolac liquid: 1 cup
0	††	114	Yogurt, plain, whole: 1 cup

Herbs, Spices, Seasonings, Etc.

Calories are negligible and need not be counted in the following list; however, many of these foods are extremely high in sodium and must be calculated very carefully.

gm. fiber	mg. chol.	mg. sodium	
0	0	250	Baking powder: 1 teaspoon
0	0	Tr.	Baking powder, low sodium: 1 teaspoon
0	0	1360	Baking soda: 1 teaspoon
††	0	10	Bakon Yeast: 1 teaspoon (12 calories)
0	0	Tr.	Bitters, Angostura: 1 teaspoon
0	0	425	Bouillon cube, beef (fat free): 1 1/2-inch cube or 4 grams
0	0	10	Bouillon cube, beef (fat free and salt free): 1 1/2-inch cube or 4 grams
0	0	5	Bouillon cube, chicken (fat free and salt free): 1 1/2-inch cube or 4 grams
Tr.	0	306	Capers: 1 tablespoon
††	0	294	Chutney: 1 tablespoon (Crosse & Blackwell's, Major Grey's)
0	0	1	Coffee: 1 cup
0	0	Tr.	Extracts: 1 teaspoon
0	0	4	Gelatin, unsweetened: 1 envelope (1 scant tablespoon)
0	0	0	Liquid smoke: 1 teaspoon
Tr.	0	63	Mustard, prepared: 1 teaspoon (French's)
Tr.	0	811	Pickles: 1 2 ounce, without sugar
0	0	6	Rennet tablets: 1 ounce
0	0	2200	Salt: 1 teaspoon
0	0	2077	Soy sauce: 1 ounce (2 tablespoons)
0	0	6	Tabasco sauce: 1/4 teaspoon
0	0	Tr.	Vinegar, cider: 1 tablespoon
0	0	5	Vinegar, red wine: 1 tablespoon
0	0	5	Vinegar, white wine: 1 tablespoon
0	0	58	Worcestershire sauce: 1 tablespoon (Lea & Perrins)

Herbs and Spices

gm. fiber	mg. chol.	mg. sodium	
.4	0	2	Allspice, ground: 1 teaspoon
.4	0	1	Allspice, whole: 1 teaspoon
††	0	Tr.	Anise seed: 1 teaspoon
.2	0	Tr.	Basil: 1 teaspoon
††	0	Tr.	Bay leaf: 1 leaf
.2	0	4	Celery seed, ground: 1 teaspoon
.2	0	2	Celery seed, whole: 1 teaspoon
††	0	31	Chili powder, seasoned: 1 teaspoon
.3	0	Tr.	Cinnamon, ground: 1 teaspoon
††	0	3	Cloves, ground: 1 teaspoon
††	0	1	Cloves, whole: 1 teaspoon
.4	0	Tr.	Coriander, ground: 1 teaspoon
.1	0	Tr.	Cumin seed: 1 teaspoon
††	0	1	Curry powder: 1 teaspoon
.4	0	Tr.	Dill seed: 1 teaspoon
††	0	Tr.	Dill weed: 1 teaspoon
.4	0	1	Fennel seed: 1 teaspoon
Tr.	0	1	Garlic powder: 1 teaspoon
††	0	1	Ginger, ground: 1 teaspoon
††	0	Tr.	Juniper berries: 1

gm. fiber	mg. chol.	mg. sodium	
††	0	Tr.	Lemon peel, dried: 1 teaspoon
††	0	Tr.	Lemon peel, fresh: 1 teaspoon
Tr.	0	2	Mace, ground: 1 teaspoon
Tr.	0	Tr.	Marjoram, dried: 1 teaspoon
Tr.	0	Tr.	Mint, dried: 1 teaspoon
††	0	Tr.	Mustard seed: 1 teaspoon
Tr.	0	Tr.	Nutmeg, ground: 1 teaspoon
.1	0	2	Onion powder: 1 teaspoon
††	0	Tr.	Oregano, dried: 1 teaspoon
.4	0	1	Paprika, ground: 1 teaspoon
.1	0	5	Parsley flakes: 1 teaspoon
.2	0	Tr.	Pepper, black: 1 teaspoon
††	0	Tr.	Pepper, cayenne: 1 teaspoon
††	0	698	Pepper, lemon: 1 teaspoon (Durkee's)
.1	0	Tr.	Pepper, white: 1 teaspoon
.2	0	Tr.	Rosemary, dried: 1 teaspoon
††	0	Tr.	Saffron, powdered: 1 teaspoon
.1	0	Tr.	Sage, dried: 1 teaspoon
.2	0	Tr.	Savory, dried: 1 teaspoon
.1	0	Tr.	Tarragon, dried: 1 teaspoon
.1	0	Tr.	Thyme, dried: 1 teaspoon
.1	0	1	Turmeric, ground: 1 teaspoon

Alcoholic Beverages

Whether you are allowed alcoholic beverages in your diet should be decided between you and your doctor. There is no question that weight loss/maintenance is simplified greatly by not drinking, as liquor of all types is high in calories. Also, as you will notice by the figures given, many alcoholic beverages are also high in sodium.

A good way to think of a cocktail, highball or glass of wine is to visualize the drink as a slice of bread with a pat of butter on it. This image may help one to refrain from having another drink more than anything else does.

There is another problem with drinking on a restricted diet. Alcohol can lead to waiting too long before eating, eating too much or eating something forbidden on the diet. Most doctors, however, consider cooking with wines completely acceptable. Wine adds very little food value to each portion, and all the alcohol is cooked away before the food is eaten.

    C=calories
    GC=grams of carbohydrates

gm. fiber	mg. chol.	mg. sodium	
0	0	17	Ale, mild, 8 oz.=98 C, 8 GC
0	0	8	Beer, 8 oz.=114 C, 11 GC

Wines

gm. fiber	mg. chol.	mg. sodium	
0	0	3	Champagne, brut, 3 oz.=75 C, 1 GC
0	0	3	Champagne, extra dry, 3 oz.= 87 C, 4 GC
0	0	4	Dubonnet, 3 oz.=96 C, 7 GC
0	0	4	Dry Marsala, 3 oz.=162 C, 18 GC
0	0	4	Sweet Marsala, 3 oz.=152 C, 23 GC
0	0	4	Muscatel, 4 oz.=158 C, 14 GC
0	0	4	Port, 4 oz.=158 C, 14 GC
0	0	4	Red wine, dry, 3 oz.=69 C, under 1 GC
0	0	4	Sake, 3 oz.=75 C, 6 GC
0	0	4	Sherry, domestic, 3½ oz.=84 C, 5 GC
0	0	4	Dry vermouth, 3½ oz.=105 C, 1 GC
0	0	4	Sweet vermouth, 3½ oz.=167 C, 12 GC
0	0	4	White wine, dry, 3 oz.=74 C, under 1 GC

Liqueurs and Cordials

gm. fiber	mg. chol.	mg. sodium	
0	0	2	Amaretto, 1 oz.=112 C, 13 GC
0	0	2	Crème de Cacao, 1 oz.=101 C, 12 GC
0	0	2	Crème de Menthe, 1 oz.=112 C, 13 GC
0	0	2	Curaçao, 1 oz.=100 C, 9 GC
0	0	2	Drambuie, 1 oz.=110 C, 11 GC
0	0	2	Tia Maria, 1 oz.=113 C, 9 GC

Spirits

Bourbon, brandy, Cognac, Canadian whiskey, gin, rye, rum, scotch, tequila and vodka are all carbohydrate free! The calories they contain depend upon the proof.

gm. fiber	mg. chol.	mg. sodium	
0	0	Tr.	80 proof, 1 oz.=67 C
0	0	Tr.	84 proof, 1 oz.=70 C
0	0	Tr.	90 proof, 1 oz.=75 C
0	0	Tr.	94 proof, 1 oz.=78 C
0	0	Tr.	97 proof, 1 oz.=81 C
0	0	Tr.	100 proof, 1 oz.=83 C

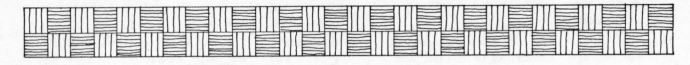

First Week Diet

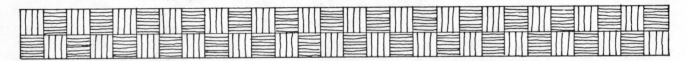

The first week of the *Fitness First* diet requires little preparation, but if you desire a more elaborate meal you may substitute one of the menus from the second week. The program starts out with an all-liquid diet of approximately 520 calories on the first day and progresses to a 700 to 800 daily calorie intake thereafter. If you wish to maintain or gain weight, increase the portion sizes. Be sure to drink eight glasses of water daily.

Day	Breakfast	Lunch	Dinner
Liquid Diet **1** 520 C.	Breakfast (131 calories) 1 serving Sunrise Special, page 87 10:30 am (25 calories) ½ cup tomato juice	Lunch (131 calories) 1 serving Banana Smoothie, page 87 3:30 pm (40 calories) ½ cup grapefruit juice	Dinner (99 calories) 1 serving White Eggnog, page 88 Bedtime (95 calories) ½ cup carrot juice
Prototype Diet **2 to 7** 700– 800 C.	Breakfast (205–225 calories) 1 low-fat or medium-fat protein portion (55–75 calories) 1 starch portion (70 calories) 1 fruit portion (40 calories) ½ non-fat milk portion (40 calories)	Lunch (285–325 calories) 2 low-fat or medium-fat protein portions (110–150 calories) 1 starch portion (70 calories) 1 vegetable portion (25 calories) 1 fruit portion (40 calories) ½ non-fat milk portion (40 calories)	Dinner (215–255 calories) 2 low-fat or medium-fat protein portions (110–150 calories) 1 vegetable portion (25 calories) 1 fruit portion (40 calories) ½ non-fat milk portion (40 calories)
2	1 soft-cooked egg 1 slice whole-wheat toast ½ cup orange juice ½ cup non-fat milk	½ cup water-packed tuna 1 slice whole-wheat toast 1 small tomato ½ cup fresh or water-packed canned pineapple chunks ½ cup non-fat milk	1 small poached chicken breast without skin 1 cup steamed broccoli, page 45 1 small fresh or water-packed canned peach ½ cup non-fat milk

Day	Breakfast	Lunch	Dinner
3	1 slice lean Canadian bacon $1/2$ English muffin $1/4$ cantaloupe $1/2$ cup non-fat milk	$1/2$ cup low-fat cottage cheese 2 graham crackers 1 cup steamed spinach, page 45 1 apple $1/2$ cup non-fat milk	3 ounces broiled fish 1 tomato 1 cup steamed green beans, page 45 $1/2$ banana $1/2$ cup non-fat milk
4	$1/4$ cup low-fat cottage cheese 1 slice whole-wheat toast 1 apple $1/2$ cup non-fat milk	2 portions (10 medium) cooked shrimp 1 slice whole-wheat toast $1/2$ cup carrot sticks or celery sticks as desired $1/2$ papaya $1/2$ cup non-fat milk	1 small broiled lean lamb chop 1 cup raw cauliflower $1/4$ cup steamed green beans, page 45 $1/2$ cup blueberries $1/2$ cup non-fat milk
5	1 soft-cooked egg 1 slice whole-wheat toast $1/2$ grapefruit $1/2$ cup non-fat milk	$1/2$ cup low-fat cottage cheese 1 slice whole-wheat toast $1/2$ cup carrot sticks 1 apple $1/2$ cup non-fat milk	1 small poached chicken breast without skin $1/2$ cup steamed snow peas, page 45 $1/2$ cup fresh or water-packed canned pineapple chunks $1/2$ cup non-fat milk
6	1 slice whole-wheat toast with 2 tablespoons un-homogenized peanut butter $1/2$ banana $1/2$ cup non-fat milk	1 small poached chicken breast without skin 1 slice whole-wheat toast 1 cup steamed or canned asparagus, page 45 $3/4$ cup strawberries $1/2$ cup non-fat milk	3 ounces poached fish 1 cup steamed okra, page 45, and $1/2$ bell pepper with $1/2$ cup tomato juice $1/4$ cantaloupe $1/2$ cup non-fat milk
7	$1/4$ cup low-fat cottage cheese $1/2$ cup cooked oatmeal with 2 tablespoons raisins $1/2$ cup non-fat milk	2 hard-cooked eggs 1 slice whole-wheat bread Lettuce as desired $1/4$ cantaloupe $1/2$ cup non-fat milk	1 small broiled filet mignon 1 cup steamed or canned asparagus, page 45 1 small tomato $1/4$ baked potato 1 small orange $1/2$ cup non-fat milk

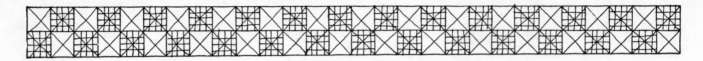

Second Week Diet

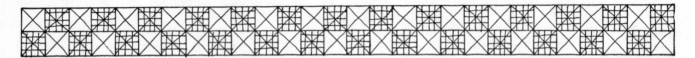

The second week takes a gourmet approach to dieting and the recipes follow. If you don't wish to take time to prepare them, you may substitute one of the menus from the first week. With the addition of one fat portion daily, this week's diet contains approximately 750 to 850 calories, except for the first day's liquid fast. Remember to continue drinking eight glasses of water daily.

Day	Breakfast	Lunch	Dinner
Liquid Diet **1** 480 C.	Breakfast (123 calories) 1 serving Coffee Carob Cooler, page 88 10:30 am (25 calories) ¹/₂ cup tomato juice	Lunch (108 calories) 1 serving Peanut Butter Punch, page 89 3:30 pm (40 calories) ¹/₂ cup grapefruit juice	Dinner (99 calories) 1 serving Paradise Punch, page 90 Bedtime (95 calories) ¹/₂ cup carrot juice
Prototype Diet **2** **to** **7** 750–850 C.	Breakfast (205–225 calories) 1 low-fat or medium-fat protein portion (55–75 calories) 1 starch portion (70 calories) 1 fruit portion (40 calories) ¹/₂ non-fat milk portion (40 calories) Plus 1 fat portion for one meal only (45 calories)	Lunch (285–325 calories) 2 low-fat or medium-fat protein portions (110–150 calories) 1 starch portion (70 calories) 1 vegetable portion (25 calories) 1 fruit portion (40 calories) ¹/₂ non-fat milk portion (40 calories)	Dinner (215–255 calories) 2 low-fat or medium-fat protein portions (110–150 calories) 1 vegetable portion (25 calories) 1 fruit portion (40 calories) ¹/₂ non-fat milk portion (40 calories)
2	1 slice Sourdough French Toast, page 53 ¹/₂ cup Strawberry Compote, page 78 ¹/₄ cup non-fat milk	1 cup Chicken Consommé, page 33 1 serving Curried Tuna Salad, page 43 1 Cinnamon Popover, page 72 1 serving Sabino Spoof with Whoopee Topping, page 75 ¹/₂ cup non-fat milk	Green salad with 2 tablespoons Skinny Italian Dressing, page 37 1 serving Italian Chicken, page 60 1 cup steamed zucchini, page 45 ¹/₂ Poached Pear in Sauterne Sauce, page 82 ¹/₂ cup non-fat milk

Day	Breakfast	Lunch	Dinner
3	1/4 cantaloupe 2 slices Canyon Ranch Bread, page 69 1/2 Dieter's Spicy Sausage patty, page 63 1/2 cup non-fat milk	1 serving Crêpes Florentine, page 55 1 apple 1/2 cup non-fat milk	1 serving Red Snapper Veracruz, page 59 1 cup steamed broccoli, page 45 1 serving Bananas North Pole, page 79 1/2 cup non-fat milk
4	1/3 cup unsweetened applesauce 1 Breakfast Pizza, page 54 1/2 cup non-fat milk	1 serving Shrimp in Papaya Cups, page 43 1/2 cup Simple Rice Salad, page 43 1/2 cup non-fat milk	1 serving Dijon Lamb Chops, page 62 1/4 cup Minted Peas, page 46 1 serving Cauliflower Incognito, page 47 1 serving Blueberry Mousse, page 81
5	1/2 grapefruit 1 Soufflé Square, page 50 1 slice whole-wheat toast 1/2 cup non-fat milk	1 serving Carrots Indienne, page 54 1 slice whole-wheat toast 1 serving Cheesecake, page 84 1/2 cup non-fat milk	1 serving Egg Flower Soup, page 34 1 serving Chinese Chicken with Snow Peas 1 serving Pineapple Boats with Coconut Sauce, page 80 1/4 cup non-fat milk
6	1 slice Banana Bread, page 70, with 2 tablespoons unhomogenized peanut butter 1/2 cup non-fat milk	1 serving Guacamole Surprise, page 39 1 serving Chicken Enchiladas, page 60 1 serving Ambrosia, page 79	1 serving Fresh Fish Gumbo, page 58 Green salad with 2 tablespoons Mystery Dressing, page 38 1 serving Melon Ball Compote, page 78 1/2 cup non-fat milk
7	1/2 cup Powerful Porridge, page 73 1/4 cup low-fat cottage cheese 1/2 cup non-fat milk	1 serving Souffle Olé, page 49 Green salad with 2 tablespoons Skinny Italian Dressing, page 37 6 Toasted Tortilla Triangles, page 72 1/4 cantaloupe 1/2 cup non-fat milk	1 serving Asparagus Vinaigrette, page 41 1 1/2 slices Steak au Poivre, page 65 1 serving Tomato Provençale, page 46 1 serving Cold Orange Soufflé, page 83 1/2 cup non-fat milk

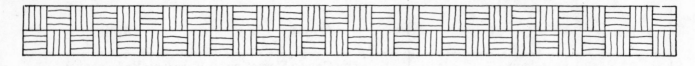

Fitness Forever Program

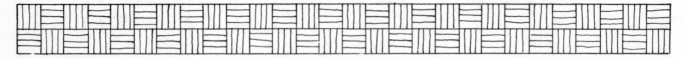

Once you have reached your desired weight and fitness level, you may increase your daily calorie intake while continuing your daily exercise program for maintaining your desired weight and level of fitness. Do not get lazy about your exercises; a lapse of a few days may bode disaster.

Watch portion sizes. The amount of food that constitutes a portion (see the food lists beginning on page 2) will probably throw you into a temporary spin. But abide by those measurements and you'll be amazed to see that you feel much better when you are less full. Eating a completely balanced meal of carefully measured portions will satisfy your hunger surprisingly well. When it becomes a habit, you'll wonder why you ever felt the need to stuff yourself.

If you have trouble eating less, there are a number of tricks to help you restrain yourself. Try the Appetite Appeaser on page 87 a half hour before mealtime; you won't be so hungry. Serve your meals on smaller plates and garnish them attractively. The portions will look less skimpy and more appealing. And remember to eat slowly. A three-pronged fork or a demitasse spoon helps reduce the amount you ingest with each bite. Finally, try some behavior modification, like always making it a rule to leave one or two bites of food on your plate.

In maintaining a diet program, most people also encounter a number of "roadblocks" that detour them from their new regimen. Dining out at restaurants or at friends' homes and the tempting array of food in the grocery store are some of the biggest roadblocks, but there are ways of circumventing them. In restaurants, order only one item—perhaps a nourishing salad—rather than the entire dinner. Most good restaurants will also "customize" your entree, if you tell them you are on a diet. For example, ask them to broil your fish rather than sautéing it in butter and serving it with a rich sauce. Friends are also understanding if you explain first that you are dieting. Make this clear when you accept a dinner invitation and give them a chance to plan a low-calorie meal for everyone. Ask for small portions when being served and simply say you don't care for dessert, instead of leaving it uneaten on your plate. Of course, do this without making your diet the focal point of the evening.

Resisting the temptations of the grocery store can be accomplished in a number of ways. Make a shopping list of those items that you truly need and promise yourself you won't impulsively add any extras to your cart. Learn to "shop the walls" of your supermarket. Here's where you will find all the fresh, nutritional foods—produce, meat and dairy products—while the junk food and fattening items hide in the inner aisles. And if your own will power isn't adequate, take a friend shopping with you with the promise that he or she will put the unnecessary items back on the shelves.

Finally, don't spend all of your time thinking of the negative aspects of dieting and dreaming of the food you can't have. Don't spend all your time on the scales, either. Instead, pay more attention to how you look and how your clothes fit you. The better you look, the easier it will become to stay that way. A skinny body with a fat, flabby middle will never make anyone think of *Fitness First.*

1500-Calorie-a-Day Diet

The following guidelines for a 1500-calorie-a-day diet are easy to follow by using the portion lists (page 2) to plan your menus. A sample menu is included to help you get started. If you find you are starting to gain weight, drop down a few calories and see what happens. If you continue to lose weight, add calories until your weight stabilizes. (Just be sure those calories are not junk food.) A member of the family who burns lots of calories either at work or by being active in sports will need more calories to keep his or her weight stabilized, but this shouldn't be too difficult to adjust.

For Each Day
2 milk portions (subtract 1 fat portion for each low-fat milk portion and 2 fat portions for each whole milk portion)
6 protein portions (subtract 1/2 fat portion for each medium-fat protein portion and 1 fat portion for each high-fat protein portion)
5 starch portions
4 fruit portions
2 vegetable portions
6 fat portions
8 Glasses of Water Each Day

Breakfast
1/2 grapefruit
1 soft-cooked egg (or equivalent in liquid egg substitute)
1 slice whole-wheat toast
1 cup non-fat milk

Lunch
1 ham and cheese sandwich on rye bread:
  1 ounce ham
  1 ounce cheese
  1 tablespoon mayonnaise
  Lettuce and tomato
  2 slices rye bread
1 apple
1 cup non-fat milk

Dinner
4 1/2 ounces broiled fish
Lettuce salad with 2 tablespoons oil and vinegar dressing
1 cup steamed broccoli with 2 teaspoons corn oil margarine
1/2 cup steamed carrots
1 small baked potato with 2 tablespoons sour cream
3/4 cup fresh strawberries with 2 teaspoons fructose

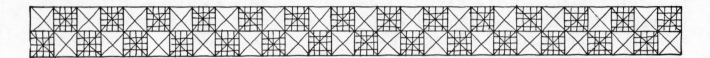

Fitting Facts

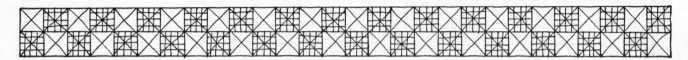

Saturated Fat Control

To lower the amount of saturated fat in your diet, apply the following rules to your diet program:
1. Use liquid vegetable oils and margarines that are high in polyunsaturated fats in place of butter. Two of the best oils for this purpose are safflower oil and corn oil.
2. Do not use coconut oil or chocolate. Many non-dairy creamers and sour-cream substitutes contain coconut oil. Use coconut extract and dry powdered cocoa.
3. Use non-fat milk, or low-sodium low-fat milk if on a low-sodium diet.
4. Avoid commercial ice cream.
5. Limit the amount of beef, lamb and pork in your diet to four or five times a week and eat fish, chicken, veal and white meat of turkey in their place.
6. Buy lean cuts of meat and trim all visible fat from them before cooking.

Cholesterol Control

To lower the amount of cholesterol in your diet, apply the following restrictions to your diet program:
1. Limit or avoid egg yolks.
2. Limit shellfish, such as oysters, clams, scallops, lobster, shrimp and crab.
3. Limit or avoid organ meats of all animals, such as liver, heart, kidney, sweetbreads and brains.

Sodium Control

1. The first and most obvious way of controlling the amount of sodium in the diet is to avoid the addition of ordinary table salt (sodium chloride), both in cooking and on the table, to already prepared foods. One teaspoon of salt contains 2,200 milligrams of sodium!
2. If you are on a sodium-restricted diet and must greatly reduce the amount of sodium in the diet, the milligrams of sodium in the serving portions of all foods can be found in the Food Lists on pages 2 through 11.

3. It is also possible to reduce sodium intake by simply using low-sodium milk in place of regular milk both for drinking and cooking.

4. *Low-sodium Baking Powder* Regular baking powder contains 40 milligrams of sodium per teaspoon, while low-sodium baking powder contains only 1 milligram per teaspoon. When using the latter, however, you will need to add half again as much (50 percent more) as you would if using regular baking powder. If you are unable to buy low-sodium baking powder, ask your druggist to make it for you, using the following formula:

Cornstarch	56.0 grams
Potassium bitartrate	112.25 grams
Potassium bicarbonate	79.5 grams
Tartaric acid	15.0 grams

5. *Potassium Bicarbonate* Potassium bicarbonate is substituted for baking soda in the low-sodium diet. The latter is sodium bicarbonate and contains 1,232 milligrams of sodium per teaspoon, while potassium bicarbonate contains no sodium. Most low-sodium cookbooks tell you to use potassium bicarbonate in the same amount as you would baking soda. It does have a definite aftertaste when used in that quantity, however. Half as much will give you the desired result in texture without the unpleasant flavor.

6. *Drinking Water* Check with your local water district about sodium content of the drinking water. If there are more than 30 milligrams of sodium per quart, it is advisable to use distilled water for both drinking and cooking.

7. To heighten flavor in the absence of added salt, fresh lemon juice in combination with a small amount of fructose and a greater amount of herbs or spices will produce the desired result.

Eggs

When using raw eggs or raw egg whites, it is important to coddle or dip the whole egg (in the shell) in boiling water for 30 seconds before using it. The reason for this is that the avedin, a component of raw egg whites, is believed to block the absorption of biotin, one of the water-soluble vitamins. Avedin is extremely sensitive to heat and coddling the egg inactivates it.

Fructose

Fructose is a natural fruit sugar that is approximately one and one-half times sweeter than sucrose (ordinary table sugar). Because of this you use less of it, therefore automatically reducing the calories. Fructose is an excellent flavor heightener in vegetable preparations when not using salt. It can also be used in small amounts in marinades even when the overall effect desired is not sweetness. This is because, in the absence of salt, fructose serves as a flavor heightener and sharpens the taste of the other ingredients.

19

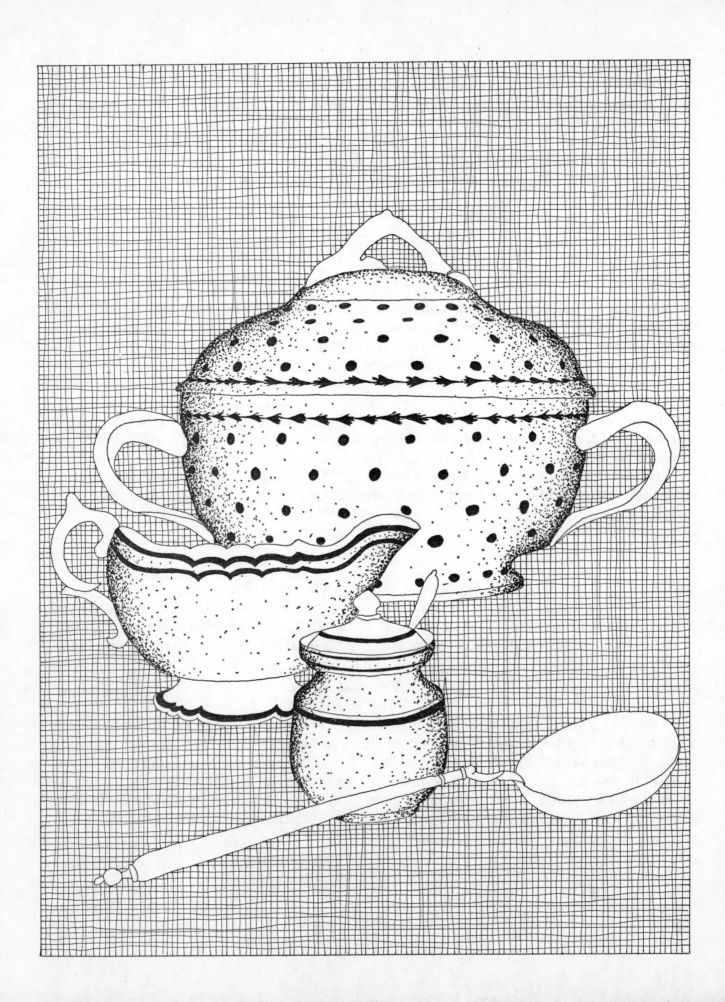

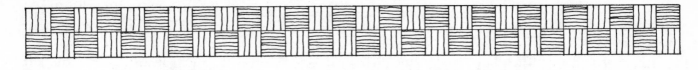

Sauces & Relishes

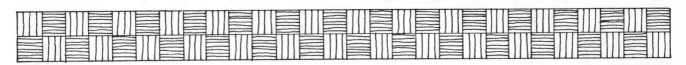

Defatted Drippings

If you love gravy but don't eat it because it's *fat, fat, fat,* then one of your problems is solved. Just defat your drippings!

All drippings are defatted in the same manner. After cooking your roast beef, leg of lamb, chicken, turkey or whatever, remove it from the roasting pan and pour the drippings into a bowl. Put the bowl in the refrigerator until the drippings are cold and all of the fat has solidified on the top. Remove the fat and you have defatted drippings.

Now, if you are in a hurry to serve your roast beef *au jus,* put the drippings in the freezer instead of the refrigerator. (Put the roast in the oven to keep it warm.) After about 20 minutes you can remove the fat, heat the *jus,* and serve.

Freeze any defatted drippings you are not using for the meal. They can be added to stocks for extra flavor and are good for making the "Skinny Gravies."

Skinny Beef Gravy

1 cup defatted beef drippings, preceding, or 1 cup concentrated beef stock
1 tablespoon cornstarch or arrowroot
2 tablespoons minced onion, browned, or 1 tablespoon dehydrated onion flakes (optional)

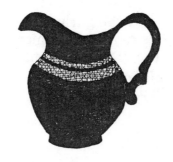

1. Heat the defatted drippings in a saucepan. As soon as they become liquid, put a little of the liquid in a cup and stir in the cornstarch or arrowroot to form a smooth paste.

2. Pour the arrowroot mixture into the saucepan, blending well.

3. Add the minced onion or onion flakes, if desired, and simmer until the gravy thickens slightly, stirring occasionally.

Note Beef Stock, page 29, can be stored in ice-cube trays in the freezer and used for individual servings of this gravy: For one serving use 2 stock "ice cubes," 1/4 teaspoon cornstarch or arrowroot and 1 teaspoon minced onion or 1/2 teaspoon dehydrated onion flakes (optional).

Makes approximately 1 cup
Free food
Calories negligible

21

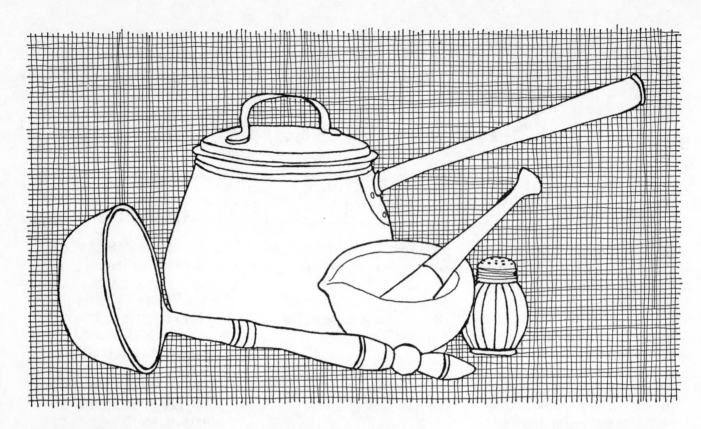

Skinny Chicken Gravy

1 cup defatted chicken
  drippings, page 21, or
1 cup concentrated
  chicken stock
1 tablespoon cornstarch or
  arrowroot
Dash garlic powder
(optional)

1. Heat the defatted drippings or stock in a saucepan. As soon as they become liquid, put a little of the liquid in a cup and stir in the cornstarch or arrowroot to form a smooth paste.

2. Pour the arrowroot mixture into the saucepan, blending in well.

3. Add the garlic powder, if desired, and simmer until the gravy thickens slightly, stirring occasionally.

Note Chicken Stock, page 30, can be stored in ice-cube trays in the freezer and used for individual servings of this gravy. For one serving use 2 Chicken Stock "ice cubes," 1/4 teaspoon cornstarch or arrowroot and garlic powder to taste (optional).

Makes approximately 1 cup
Free food
Calories negligible

Skinny Turkey Gravy

2 cups defatted turkey
 drippings, page 21
2 tablespoons cornstarch
 or arrowroot
1/2 cup minced green onion
 tops (optional)
1/2 cup chopped fresh
 mushrooms (optional)
2 tablespoons minced
 parsley (optional)

1. Heat the defatted drippings in a saucepan. As soon as they become liquid, put a little of the liquid in a cup and stir in the cornstarch or arrowroot to form a smooth paste.

2. Pour the arrowroot mixture back into the saucepan, blending in well.

3. Add the green onion tops, mushrooms and/or parsley, if desired, and simmer until the gravy thickens slightly, stirring occasionally.

Makes approximately 2 cups
Free food
Calories negligible

Skinny Giblet Gravy

2 cups defatted Turkey
 Giblet Stock, page 32, or
 Chicken Giblet Stock,
 page 31
2 tablespoons cornstarch
 or arrowroot
1/2 cup minced green onion
 tops (optional)
1/2 cup chopped fresh
 mushrooms (optional)
2 tablespoons minced
 parsley (optional)
1 or 2 cups chopped
 cooked giblets

1. Heat the defatted Giblet Stock in a saucepan. As soon as it becomes liquid, put a little of the liquid in a cup and stir in the cornstarch or arrowroot to form a smooth paste.

2. Pour the arrowroot mixture back into the saucepan, blending in well.

3. Add the green onion tops, mushrooms and/or parsley and simmer until the gravy thickens slightly, stirring occasionally. Add the giblets and heat through.

Makes 4 servings
Each serving with 1/4 cup giblets
contains approximately:
    1 low-fat protein portion
    55 calories

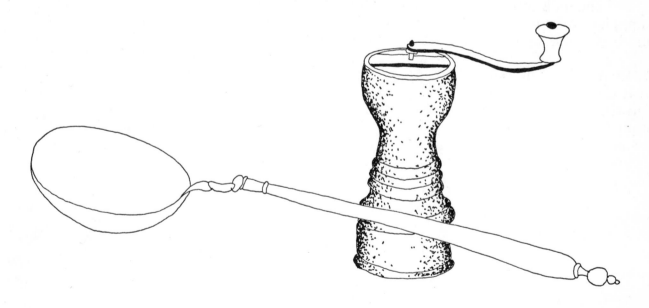

23

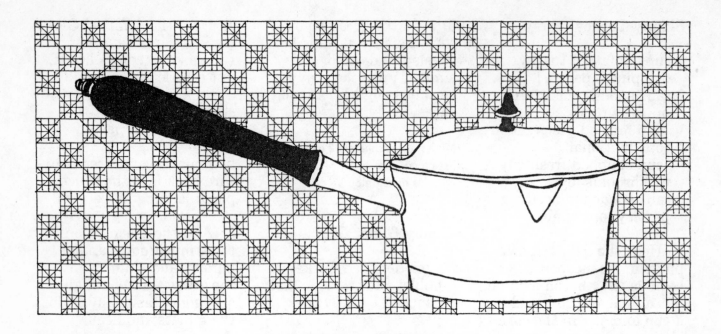

White Sauce

2 cups non-fat milk
1 tablespoon corn oil
  margarine
2½ tablespoons sifted
  all-purpose flour
⅛ teaspoon salt

1. Put the milk in a sauce-pan, place over low heat and bring to a simmer.

2. In another saucepan, melt the margarine and add the flour, stirring constantly. Cook, stirring, for 3 minutes. *Do not brown.*

3. Remove the flour-margarine mixture from the heat and add the simmering milk all at once, stirring constantly with a wire whisk.

4. Put the sauce on low heat and cook slowly for 20 minutes, stirring occasionally. If you wish a thicker sauce, cook a little longer.

5. Add the salt and mix thoroughly. If there are lumps in the sauce (though there shouldn't be any by this method), whirl it in a blender container until smooth.

Makes 1½ cups
¾ cup contains approximately:
  1½ fat portions
  ½ starch portion
  1 non-fat milk portion
  183 calories
1½ cups contain approximately:
  3 fat portions
  1 starch portion
  2 non-fat milk portions
  365 calories

Cheddar Cheese Sauce

1½ cups White Sauce,
   preceding
½ cup non-fat milk
⅛ teaspoon ground white
   pepper
¼ teaspoon dry mustard
½ cup grated sharp
   Cheddar cheese

1. Place the White Sauce
on low heat and add the
milk, pepper, dry mustard
and grated cheese, blend-
ing in well.

2. Heat, stirring, until the
cheese is completely
melted.

Makes 2 cups
1 cup contains approximately:
   1½ fat portions
    ½ starch portion
     1 non-fat milk portion
     1 high-fat protein portion
   278 calories
2 cups contain approximately:
    3 fat portions
    1 starch portion
    2 non-fat milk portions
    2 high-fat protein portions
   555 calories

Mornay Sauce

1½ cups White Sauce,
   preceding
½ cup non-fat milk
½ cup grated Gruyère or
   Swiss cheese
⅛ teaspoon ground
   nutmeg
⅛ teaspoon ground white
   pepper

1. Place the White Sauce
on low heat and add the
milk, cheese, nutmeg and
pepper, blending in
well.

2. Heat, stirring, until
the cheese is completely
melted.

Variation Substitute
½ cup Chicken Stock,
page 30, for the ½ cup
non-fat milk.

Makes 2 cups
1 cup contains approximately:
   1½ fat portions
    ½ starch portion
   1¼ non-fat milk portions
    1 high-fat protein portion
   298 calories
2 cups contain approximately:
    3 fat portions
    1 starch portion
   2½ non-fat milk portions
    2 high-fat protein portions
   596 calories

Jelled Milk

1 envelope (1 tablespoon)
   unflavored gelatin
2 tablespoons cold water
¼ cup water, boiling
1 cup non-fat milk

1. Soften the gelatin in the
cold water.

2. Add the boiling water
and stir until the gelatin is
completely dissolved.

3. Add the milk and mix
well.

4. Place the gelatin-milk
mixture in a covered con-
tainer in the refrigerator.
When it is jelled, it is
ready to use.

5. To serve, mix jelled
milk with an equal amount
of non-fat milk in the
blender and use over fruit
or cereal. The thick,
creamy consistency makes
the milk seem richer.

Makes 1 cup
1 cup contains approximately:
    1 non-fat milk portion
    80 calories

Teriyaki Marinade

1³/4 cups soy sauce
3 tablespoons fructose
2 cloves garlic, crushed
1 tablespoon grated
   ginger root, or ¹/2 teaspoon ground ginger

1. Combine all of the ingredients and store in the
refrigerator for 1 day
before using.

2. Marinate chicken,
beef or pork for 2 hours,
and fish and shellfish for
1 hour, then broil or barbe-
cue over charcoal.

Note   Use ground ginger
only if you *absolutely* can't
find the fresh. Fresh ginger
makes all the difference in
the world in taste. If
ginger root is sometimes
difficult to find in your
area, buy a quantity of it
when it is available and
store it, sealed in a plastic
bag, in the freezer.

This marinade can also be
used as a sauce to serve
with barbecued meats and
seafood. Calories need not
be counted if using as a
marinade, but must be
counted when serving as a
sauce.

1 recipe contains approximately:
   3 fruit portions
   120 calories

Seafood Cocktail Sauce

1 cup Tomato Juice Cat-
   sup, following
1 tablespoon fresh lemon
   juice
1 teaspoon prepared horse-
   radish, or to taste

1. Combine all of the ingredients and chill well.

2. Serve over cold cooked
shrimp, crab, lobsters or a
combination, or on raw
oysters or clams.

Makes 1 cup
2 tablespoons contain approximately:
   ¹/4 vegetable portion
   7 calories

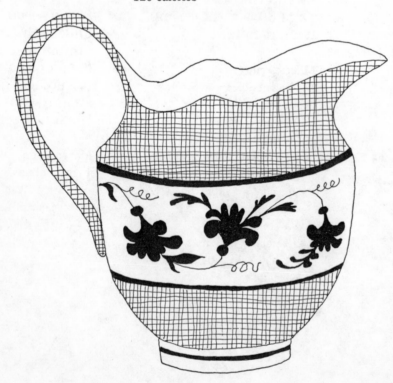

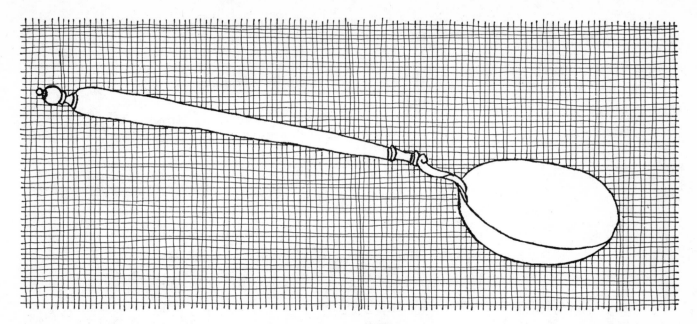

Fresh Cranberry Relish

2 small oranges
2/3 cup fructose
1 pound (4 cups) fresh
  cranberries

1. Wash the oranges well and grate 2 tablespoons of the peel. Be careful to grate only the orange-colored part, or zest.

2. Peel the oranges and cut them in pieces, removing the seeds and connecting membranes.

3. Put the orange pieces, grated peel and fructose in a blender container and mix well.

4. With the blender motor running, add the cranberries, a few at a time. Don't blend the mixture too finely as you want a fairly coarse relish.

5. Store in a covered container in the refrigerator. Make the relish several days before you plan to serve it to allow the flavors to blend.

Makes 4 cups
1/2 cup contains approximately:
  1 1/2 fruit portions
  60 calories

Tomato Juice Catsup

1 quart tomato juice
1/4 cup wine vinegar
2 cloves garlic
3/4 teaspoon fructose

1. Put the tomato juice, vinegar and garlic in a saucepan and bring to a boil.

2. Reduce the heat to very low and simmer, uncovered, for about 2 1/2 hours, or until the mixture is of desired thickness.

3. Remove from the heat and cool to room temperature. Remove and discard the garlic cloves; stir in the fructose.

4. Store in the refrigerator in a covered glass or plastic container.

Makes about 1 1/2 cups
2 tablespoons contain approximately:
  1/4 vegetable portion
  7 calories

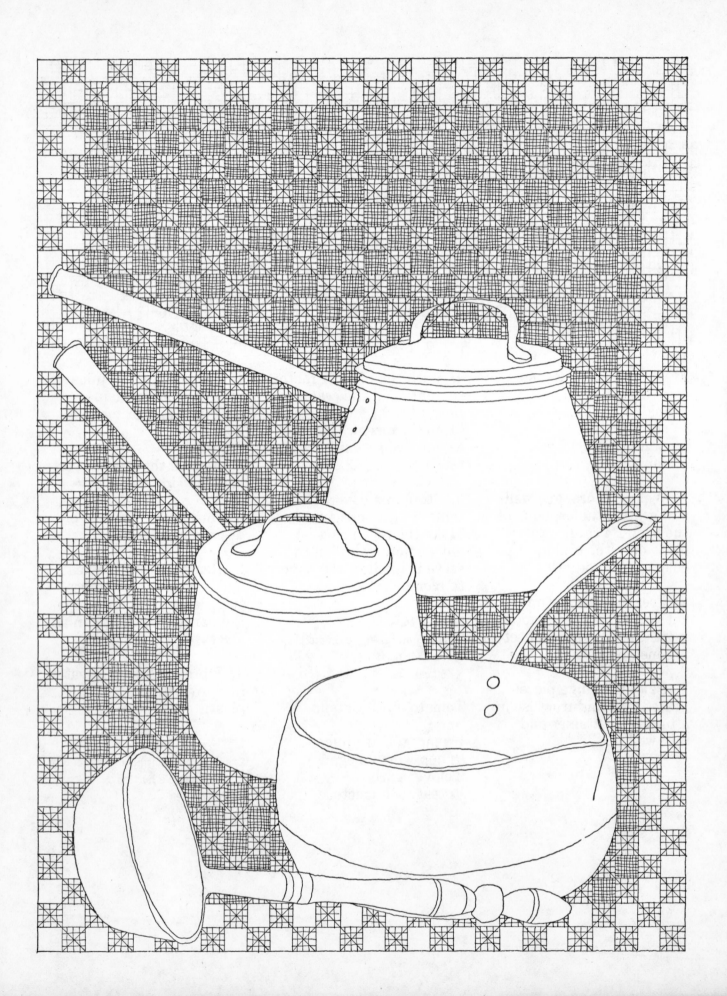

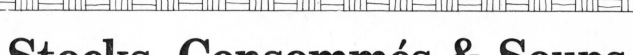

Stocks, Consommés & Soups

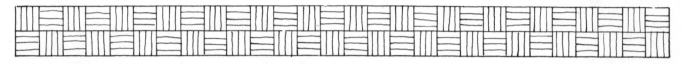

Beef Stock

3 pounds beef or veal bones
1 pound meat, cut of choice
 (optional)
2 carrots, scraped and cut
 into pieces
2 stalks celery, without
 leaves
1 onion, cut in half
1 tomato, cut in half
3 cloves garlic
2 parsley sprigs
2 whole cloves
1/4 teaspoon crumbled dried
 thyme
1/4 teaspoon crumbled dried
 marjoram
1 bay leaf
10 peppercorns
1 teaspoon salt
Defatted beef drippings,
 page 21 (optional)

1. Put the bones and enough cold water to cover by 1 inch in a large soup kettle. Bring to a boil.

2. Simmer slowly for 5 minutes, then remove and discard any residue that has formed on the surface.

3. Add the meat, vegetables and spices and enough additional cold water to cover by 1 inch.

4. Cover, leaving the lid ajar about 1 inch to allow the steam to escape. Simmer very slowly for at least 5 hours. (Ten hours are even better.)

5. When the stock is finished cooking, strain it and allow it to come to room temperature. Refrigerate, uncovered, overnight. The next morning remove and discard the fat that has hardened on the surface.

6. After removing every bit of fat, warm the stock until it becomes liquid. Strain the liquid and add salt to taste. If the flavor is too weak, boil it to evaporate more of the water and concentrate the strength.

7. Store the stock in the freezer, putting some of it in ice-cube trays for individual servings (2 cubes= 1/4 cup). The stock may also be stored in a tightly covered container for not more than 2 days in the refrigerator.

Makes about 2 1/2 quarts (10 cups)
Free food
Calories negligible

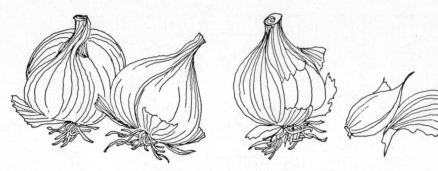

Chicken Stock

3 pounds chicken parts
(wings, backs, etc.)
1 whole stewing chicken
(optional)
2 carrots, scraped and cut
into pieces
2 stalks celery, without
leaves
1 onion, cut in half
2 cloves garlic
1 bay leaf
1/4 teaspoon crumbled dried
basil
8 peppercorns
1 teaspoon salt

1. Put the chicken parts
and whole chicken, if used,
in a large soup kettle. Add
cold water to cover by 1
inch and bring to a boil.

2. Simmer slowly for 5
minutes, then remove and
discard any residue that
has formed on the surface.

3. Add all of the remaining
ingredients and cover, leaving the lid ajar about 1
inch to allow steam to
escape. Simmer very slowly
for 3 hours or until the
chicken is tender.

4. Remove the chicken and
continue to simmer the
stock for 3 or 4 hours
longer. (If desired, bone the
chicken and return the
bones to the pot. Use the
meat in any dish requiring
cooked chicken.)

5. When the stock is fin-
ished cooking, strain it and
allow it to come to room
temperature. Refrigerate it,
uncovered, overnight. The
next morning, remove and
discard the fat that has
hardened on the surface.

6. After removing every
bit of fat, warm the stock
until it becomes liquid.
Strain the liquid and add
salt to taste. If the flavor
is too weak, boil it to evaporate more of the water
and concentrate the
strength.

7. Store the stock in the
freezer, putting some of it
in ice-cube trays for in-
dividual servings (2 cubes
=1/4 cup). The stock may
also be stored in a tightly
covered container for not
more than 2 days in the
refrigerator.

Makes about 2 1/2 quarts (10 cups)
Free food
Calories negligible

Chicken Giblet Stock

Hearts, gizzards, livers
   and necks from
   2 or 3 chickens
1 stalk celery, cut into
   pieces
1 carrot, scraped and cut
   into pieces
1 onion, cut into quarters
2 bay leaves
1/4 teaspoon crumbled dried
   basil
1 teaspoon salt
4 peppercorns

1. Put all of the ingredients in a large saucepan with enough cold water to cover by 1 inch. Bring to a boil.

2. Simmer slowly for 5 minutes, then remove and discard any residue that has formed on the surface.

3. Cover, leaving the lid ajar about 1 inch to allow steam to escape. Simmer very slowly for 3 hours.

4. When the stock is finished cooking, strain it, discarding the vegetables. Chop the giblets, cover and refrigerate. Allow the stock to come to room temperature, then refrigerate it, uncovered, overnight. The next morning, remove and discard the fat that has hardened on the surface.

5. After removing every bit of fat, warm the stock until it becomes liquid. Strain the liquid and add salt to taste. If the flavor is too weak, boil it to evaporate more of the water and concentrate the strength.

6. Return the chopped giblets to the pot, if desired, and heat through.

Note This stock is delicious served over steamed rice. Add the giblets to the stock and make it a complete meal (1 cup chopped giblets= 4 low-fat protein portions).

Makes 1 1/2 to 2 quarts (6 to 8 cups)
Free food
Calories negligible

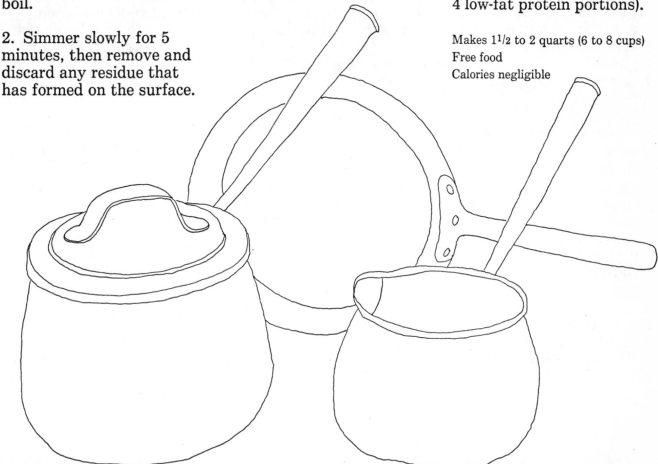

31

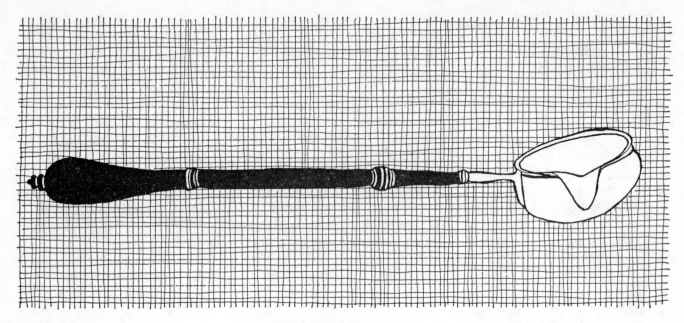

Turkey Giblet Stock

Heart, gizzard, liver and
   neck from 1 turkey
1 stalk celery, cut into
   pieces
1 onion, cut into quarters
1 clove garlic
1 bay leaf
1/4 teaspoon crumbled dried
   basil
1/8 teaspoon crumbled dried
   thyme
1/8 teaspoon crumbled dried
   marjoram
1 teaspoon salt
4 peppercorns
Defatted turkey drippings,
   page 21 (optional)

1. Put all of the ingre-
dients in a large saucepan
with enough cold water to
cover by 1 inch. Bring to a
boil.

2. Simmer slowly for 5
minutes, then remove and
discard any residue that
has formed on the surface.

3. Cover, leaving the lid
ajar about 1 inch to allow
steam to escape. Simmer
very slowly for 3 hours.

4. When the stock is fin-
ished cooking, strain it,
discarding the vegetables.
Chop the giblets, including
the lean meat on the neck,
cover and refrigerate.
Allow the stock to come to
room temperature, then
refrigerate it, uncovered,
overnight. The next morn-
ing, remove and discard
the fat that has hardened
on the surface.

5. After removing every
bit of fat, warm the stock
until it becomes liquid.
Strain the liquid and add
salt to taste. If the flavor
is too weak, boil it to
evaporate more of the
water and concentrate the
strength.

6. Return the chopped giblets to the pot, if desired,
and heat through.

Note This stock is delicious served over steamed
rice. Add the giblets to
the stock and make it a
complete meal (1 cup
chopped giblets=4 low-fat
protein portions).

Makes 11/2 to 2 quarts (6 to 8 cups)
Free food
Calories negligible

32

Chicken Consommé

4 egg whites
2 quarts (8 cups) Chicken
    Stock, page 30
2 bay leaves
2 sprigs parsley
4 green onion tops, chopped
2 carrots, chopped
Salt to taste
2 envelopes (2 tablespoons)
    unflavored gelatin (op-
    tional)

1. Beat the egg whites
with a wire whisk until
they are slightly foamy.

2. Add 2 cups of the cold
stock to the egg whites
and beat together lightly.

3. Put the remaining 6
cups of stock in a saucepan
with all of the other ingredients, bring to a boil and
remove from the heat.

4. Slowly pour the egg
white–stock mixture into
the hot stock, stirring with
the wire whisk as you do.

5. Put the saucepan back
on very low heat and stir
gently until it starts to
simmer. Put the pan half
on the heat and half off so
that it is barely simmering
and turn the pan around
every few minutes. Simmer
for 40 minutes.

6. Let the consommé cool
slightly. Line a colander or
a strainer with 2 or 3
layers of damp cheesecloth
and ladle the consommé
through the cheesecloth.
Allow it to drain undis-
turbed until it has all
seeped through.

Makes 2 quarts (8 cups)
Free food
Calories negligible

Consommé Madrilène

3 large ripe tomatoes, sliced
2 stalks celery, chopped
1 leek, white part only,
    chopped
1 carrot, sliced
1 onion, sliced
1 teaspoon fresh lemon
    juice
6 peppercorns
2 quarts (8 cups) Chicken
    Stock, page 30
2 bay leaves
2 envelopes (2 tablespoons)
    unflavored gelatin
1/4 cup cold water
Salt and freshly ground
    black pepper to taste
2 drops red food coloring
    (optional)

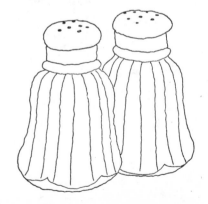

1. Place all of the ingredients in a large pot or
soup kettle, except the
gelatin, water, salt and
pepper and food coloring,
and bring to a boil.

2. Reduce the heat and
cover, leaving the lid ajar
about 1 inch to allow
steam to escape. Simmer
slowly for 2 hours.

3. Soften the gelatin in the
water and add to the hot
consommé, stirring over
low heat with a wire whisk
until completely dissolved.

4. Cool slightly and strain
through a fine strainer.

5. Season to taste with
salt and pepper. Add the
red food coloring, if
desired, for better color.

6. Cool to room tempera-
ture and refrigerate. When
the consommé is completely
jelled, unmold and cut off
and discard the part con-
taining the sediment. Cut
up the clear part and serve
in chilled glasses or cups
or in Artichoke Bowls.

Makes 1 to 1 1/2 quarts (4 to 6 cups)
Free food
Calories negligible

Cold Consommé with Mushrooms

1/4 cup fresh lemon juice
1 cup thinly sliced fresh mushrooms (1/4 pound)
2 cups Consommé Madrilène, page 33, or beef consommé, cold
4 tablespoons plain low-fat yogurt
5 teaspoons caviar

1. Pour the lemon juice over the mushrooms and refrigerate them for at least 2 hours.

2. Add the mushrooms to the consommé and mix well.

3. Put the consommé in 4 chilled bowls or icers. Put 1 tablespoon of yogurt on top of each one and 1 1/4 teaspoons of caviar on top of each spoonful of yogurt.

Makes 4 servings
Each serving contains approximately:
   1/4 medium-fat protein portion
   19 calories

Egg Flower Soup

6 cups Chicken Stock, page 30
4 eggs
1/4 cup chopped chives or green onion tops

1. Bring the stock to a boil in a saucepan.

2. Beat the eggs until they are frothy.

3. Slowly pour the eggs into the boiling stock, stirring constantly with a fork.

4. Continue to stir the soup rapidly until the egg sets and forms long thin strands.

5. Ladle into 8 bowls and sprinkle each with chives or green onion tops. Serve very hot.

Makes 8 servings
Each serving contains approximately:
   1/2 medium-fat protein portion
   38 calories

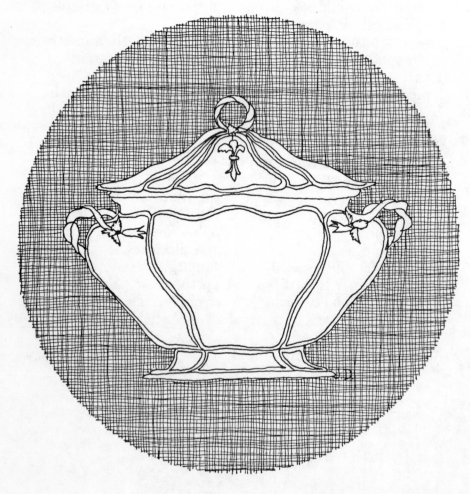

Sherried Pea Soup

2 cups green peas
   (2 pounds unshelled)
1 cup Chicken Stock,
   page 30
1/8 teaspoon white pepper
1 cup non-fat milk
1/4 cup dry sherry
1/2 teaspoon freshly grated
   lemon peel

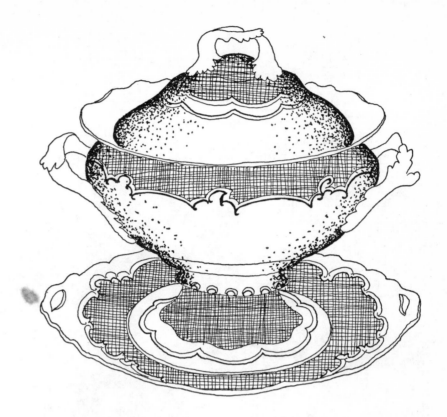

1. Combine the peas, stock and white pepper in a saucepan. Bring to a boil, cover and cook until the peas are just tender, about 5 minutes.

2. Cool the peas slightly and put them into a blender container. Add the milk and sherry and blend until smooth.

3. Transfer the soup to a container, cover and chill thoroughly.

4. Serve in chilled bowls or in icers and sprinkle each serving with a pinch of lemon peel.

Note This soup may also be served hot.

Makes 4 servings
Each serving contains approximately:
   2 vegetable portions
   1/4 non-fat milk portion
   70 calories

Cold Curried Orange Soup

2 cups fresh orange juice
2 tablespoons quick-cooking
   tapioca
1 teaspoon fructose
1/4 teaspoon curry powder
1/8 teaspoon ground ginger
1/4 cup plain non-fat
   yogurt

1. Combine all of the ingredients, except the yogurt, in a saucepan and allow to stand for 5 minutes.

2. Put the pan on medium heat and bring the mixture to a boil, stirring constantly.

3. As soon as it comes to a boil, remove the pan from the heat and cool to room temperature.

4. Cover and chill thoroughly. Just before serving, stir in the yogurt, mixing thoroughly. Serve in chilled bowls or in icers.

Makes 4 servings
Each serving contains approximately:
   1 1/2 fruit portions
   60 calories

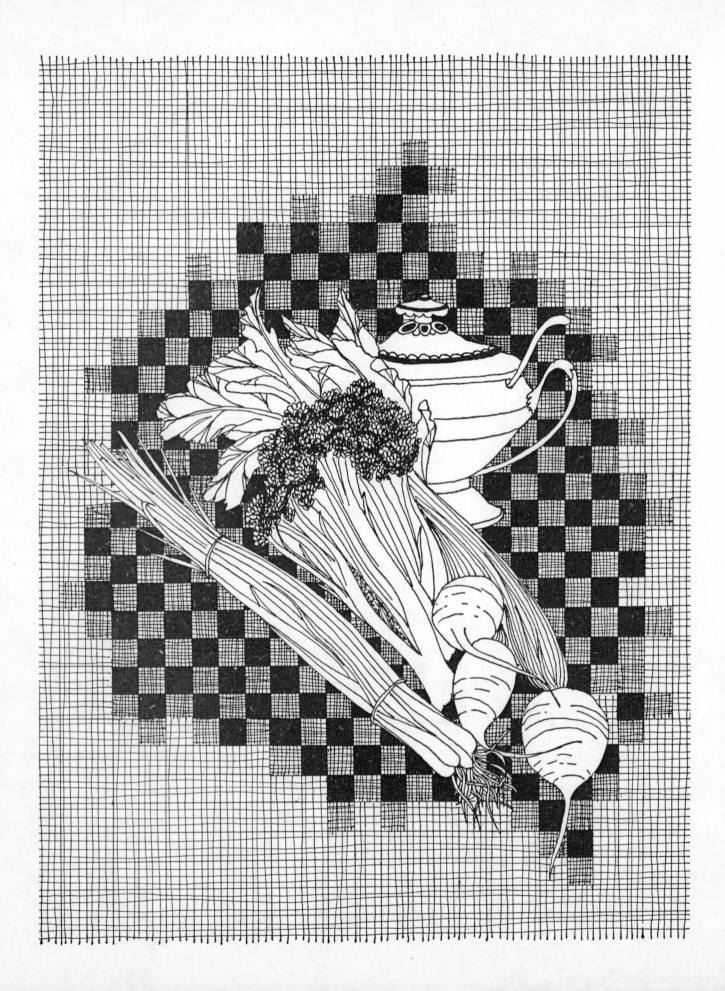

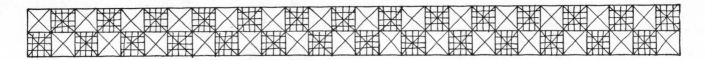

Salads & Vegetables

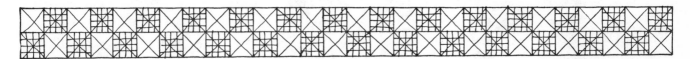

Skinny Italian Dressing

One 16-ounce can tomatoes,
undrained (2 cups)
2 tablespoons fresh lemon
juice
2 tablespoons red-wine
vinegar
1 teaspoon crumbled dried
oregano
1/2 teaspoon crumbled dried
basil
1/2 teaspoon crumbled dried
tarragon
1/2 teaspoon fructose
1/4 teaspoon garlic powder
1/4 teaspoon onion powder
1/4 teaspoon freshly ground
black pepper

1. Put all of the ingre-
dients in a blender con-
tainer and blend until
smooth.

2. Store in the refrigerator
in a covered container.

Makes 2 1/2 cups
2 tablespoons contain approximately:
Free food
Calories negligible

Canyon Ranch Dressing

1 1/2 teaspoons salt
1/4 cup red-wine vinegar
1 teaspoon fructose
1/4 teaspoon freshly ground
black pepper
1/4 teaspoon garlic powder
1 1/2 teaspoons crumbled
dried oregano
1 teaspoon crumbled dried
basil
1 teaspoon crumbled dried
tarragon
2 teaspoons fresh lemon
juice
1 teaspoon Worcester-
shire sauce
1/4 teaspoon Dijon-style
mustard
1/2 cup water
2 tablespoons corn oil

1. Dissolve the salt in the
vinegar, then add all of the
remaining ingredients, except the oil, and mix well.

2. Slowly stir in the oil.
Pour into a jar with a
tightly fitting lid and
shake vigorously for 1 full
minute.

3. Store in a covered container in the refrigerator.

Makes 1 cup
2 tablespoons contain approximately:
3/4 fat portion
34 calories

Curried Yogurt Dressing

1 cup (1/2 pint) plain low-fat
yogurt
2 tablespoons sour cream
3/4 teaspoon curry powder
1/4 teaspoon ground ginger
1/2 teaspoon coconut extract

1. Put all of the ingre-
dients in a bowl and mix
thoroughly.

2. Store in the refrigerator
in a covered container.

Makes 1 cup
1/4 cup contains approximately:
1/4 low-fat milk portion
1/4 fat portion
31 calories

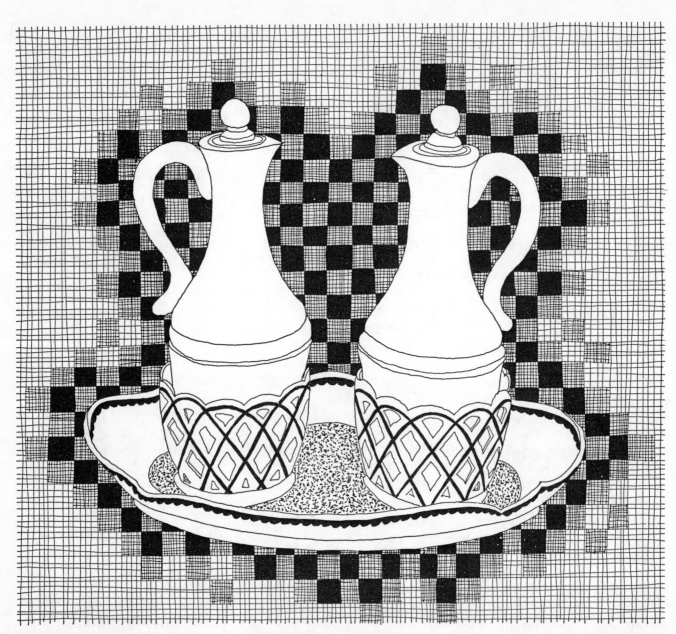

Mystery Dressing

3/4 cup unsweetened pine-
    apple juice
3/4 cup tomato juice
1 tablespoon fresh lemon
    juice
1/4 teaspoon fructose
1/4 teaspoon salt
1 clove garlic, pressed
1/8 teaspoon freshly ground
    black pepper

1/8 teaspoon dry mustard
1 tablespoon chopped
    pimiento
1 teaspoon capers, chopped

1. Combine the pineapple
juice, tomato juice, lemon
juice, fructose and salt,
stirring until the salt is
completely dissolved.

2. Add all of the remaining
ingredients and mix
thoroughly.

3. Store in a tightly
covered container in the
refrigerator.

Makes 1 1/2 cups
2 tablespoons contain approximately:
Free food
Calories negligible

38

Marinated Mushrooms

One 8-ounce can button
mushrooms
2 cloves garlic, halved
2 tablespoons olive oil
4 teaspoons red-wine
vinegar
1 teaspoon Worcester-
shire sauce
1/8 teaspoon salt

1. Open and drain the
mushrooms, reserving the
liquid.

2. Place half of the mushrooms in a glass jar with a
tightly fitting lid and put
one of the split garlic
cloves on top of them.

3. Add the remaining
mushrooms and put the re-
maining halved garlic clove
on top.

4. Combine all of the re-
maining ingredients, in-
cluding the reserved can liquid, and pour over the
mushrooms.

5. Cover the jar and shake
to mix well. Refrigerate for
24 hours before serving.

6. Serve as an hors
d'oeuvre. Put a toothpick
in each mushroom and
serve on a plate or in a
shallow bowl.

Variation   Substitute 1
cup fresh button mush-
rooms for the canned.
Blanch the fresh mush-
rooms in 1 cup chicken
stock for 1 to 2 minutes.
Drain, reserving the stock.
Proceed as directed in the
recipe, substituting the
chicken stock for the can
liquid.

Makes 1 cup
1/4 cup contains approximately:
    1/2 vegetable exchange
    13 calories

Guacamole Surprise

8 lettuce leaves
1 pound asparagus spears
1 tablespoon fresh lemon
juice
1 1/2 tablespoons finely
chopped onion
1 medium tomato, chopped
1 teaspoon salt
1/4 teaspoon ground cumin
1/4 teaspoon chili powder
1/8 teaspoon garlic powder
Dash Tabasco sauce
1/2 cup sour cream
1 envelope (1 tablespoon)
unflavored gelatin
1/4 cup cold water
8 small tomato wedges for
garnish

1. Wash and dry the let-
tuce leaves and put them
in the refrigerator to chill.

2. Wash the asparagus
and break off the tough
ends. Cut the spears into
1-inch pieces and steam until just fork tender, about
4 minutes. Cool the asparagus to room temperature.

3. Put the asparagus and
all the remaining ingredients, except the gelatin,
water and tomato wedges,
in a blender container and
blend until smooth. Leave
the mixture in the con-
tainer.

4. Put the gelatin in a
small saucepan, add water
and let stand for 5 min-
utes. Place the pan on low
heat and cook, stirring constantly, until the gelatin is
completely dissolved. *Do
not allow it to come to a
boil.*

5. Add the dissolved gelatin to the blender container
and blend on low speed until thoroughly mixed. Pour
the mixture into a bowl
and chill until firm.

6. Spoon an equal-sized
portion of the mixture on
each of the chilled lettuce
leaves. Garnish with
tomato wedges.

Makes 8 servings
Each serving contains approximately:
    1/2 fat portion
    1/2 vegetable portion
    36 calories

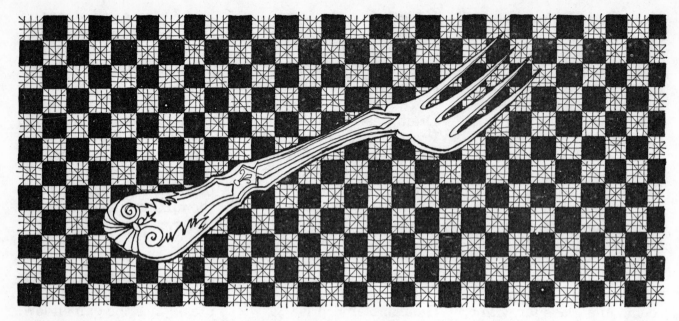

Artichoke Bowls

Artichokes, any number
    desired
2 cloves garlic, halved
1 thick lemon slice
1/2 teaspoon salt
Canyon Ranch Dressing,
    page 37

1. Wash the artichokes
well and pull off the tough
outer leaves.

2. Holding each artichoke
by its stem, cut the tips off
the leaves with scissors.
When trimming the tips,
start at the bottom of the
artichoke and work your
way to the top in a spiral
pattern. Trim off the stem
even with the base, turn
the artichoke upside down
and press firmly to open it
up as much as possible.

2. Pour water to a depth
of 2 inches in the bottom
of a saucepan. Add the
garlic, lemon slice and salt
and bring to a boil.

4. Place the artichokes in
the boiling water, cover
tightly and cook over
medium heat about
40 minutes or until the
stem ends can be easily
pierced with a fork.

5. Remove the artichokes
from the water and place
upside down to drain until
cool enough to handle easily.
Remove the center leaves
and spread the artichokes
open very carefully. Reach
down into the center and
remove the furry choke,
pulling it out a little at a
time. A grapefruit spoon
works well to remove any
hard-to-reach choke.

6. Place the artichokes
right side up in a glass
baking dish. Pour a little
Canyon Ranch Dressing
into each and chill several
hours before serving.

Note   You can serve soup
and salad together as a
first course. Place the
chilled Artichoke Bowl on
a plate, fill with Consommé
Madrilène and top with
1 tablespoon sour cream
and 1/2 teaspoon caviar. On
the side, heap 1 tablespoon
of sour cream as a dip for
the leaves. First, you eat
your soup out of your
"bowl" and then you eat
the "bowl" for your salad.

1 artichoke without dressing
contains approximately:
    1 vegetable portion
    25 calories

40

Shades of Green Salad

3 large cucumbers
1 tablespoon fructose
1/2 cup fresh lemon juice
1/4 cup finely chopped fresh
　　mint leaves
Mint sprigs for garnish

1. Peel the cucumbers and cut them in half lengthwise. Remove all of the seeds from each cucumber half, using a melon-ball cutter or a teaspoon.

2. Slice each cucumber half crosswise into very thin slices.

3. Spread the cucumber slices out in a large glass baking dish and sprinkle the fructose evenly over the top. Cover and let stand for at least 2 hours.

4. Drain the cucumber slices thoroughly and set aside.

5. Combine the lemon juice and chopped mint and mix thoroughly. Add the cucumber slices, again mixing thoroughly.

6. Serve on chilled plates and garnish each serving with a sprig of mint.

Makes 8 servings
Each serving contains approximately:
Free food
Calories negligible

Cold Pea Salad

3 cups green peas
　　(3 pounds unshelled)
1 cup (1/2 pint) sour cream
1 cup finely chopped green
　　onion tops
1 teaspoon seasoned salt

1. Steam the peas until crisp tender, then cool.

2. Mix together the sour cream, green onion tops and seasoned salt.

3. Fold the sour cream mixture into the cooled green peas, cover and refrigerate for 2 days before serving.

Variations Two 10-ounce packages frozen peas may be substituted for the fresh. To cut the fat portions in half, substitute 1/2 cup plain low-fat yogurt mixed with 1/2 cup sour cream for the 1 cup sour cream.

Makes 6 servings
Each serving contains approximately:
　　1 vegetable portion
　　2 1/2 fat portions
　　138 calories

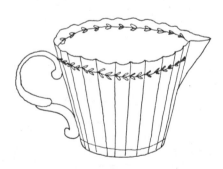

Asparagus Vinaigrette

40 asparagus spears
1 cup Canyon Ranch
　　Dressing, page 37
One 4-ounce jar whole
　　pimientos, cut into
　　julienne
1/4 cup capers

1. Wash the asparagus and break off the tough ends. Steam for about 8 minutes, or until tender.

2. Cool the asparagus to room temperature and place in a glass baking dish with all the tips pointing in the same direction (this makes removing them for serving much simpler). Pour the dressing over the asparagus and cover the dish tightly with foil.

3. Refrigerate all day or overnight to thoroughly marinate the asparagus.

4. To serve, divide the asparagus among 8 chilled asparagus dishes or salad plates and arrange an equal amount of pimiento strips and capers over each serving.

Makes 8 servings
Each serving contains approximately:
　　1/2 vegetable portion
　　1/2 fat portion
　　36 calories

Hawaiian Cole Slaw

One 20-ounce can crushed
  pineapple in natural juice,
  undrained
1 teaspoon fructose
1½ teaspoons coconut
  extract
1 head cauliflower, finely
  grated (about 4 cups)
Ground cinnamon
Mint sprigs for garnish
  (optional)

1. Pour the juice off the
pineapple into a large bowl
and set the crushed pine-
apple aside to add later.

2. Add the fructose and
coconut extract to the
juice and mix until the
fructose is thoroughly
dissolved.

3. Add the cauliflower to
the juice and mix well.
Add the crushed pineapple
and mix well again.

4. Cover and refrigerate
for at least 2 hours before
serving. (It is even better
if allowed to stand several
hours or overnight.)

5. Divide evenly onto
chilled plates and lightly
sprinkle each serving with
cinnamon. Garnish with a
mint sprig, if available.

Variation This salad is
also good with the addition
of diced apples or oranges,
sliced bananas, chopped
mangoes or papayas, or
practically any fresh fruit
you desire. You can also
add a variety of fruit and
serve it in sherbet glasses
as a dessert instead of a
salad. Or add tuna or diced
cooked chicken or turkey
and serve as a luncheon
entree.

Makes 6 servings
Each serving contains approximately:
  1 fruit portion
  40 calories

Tabbouli

1 cup cracked wheat
  (bulgur)
¼ cup fresh lemon juice
½ teaspoon salt
¼ teaspoon freshly ground
  black pepper
1 clove garlic, minced
1 tablespoon water
3 tablespoons olive oil
2 tomatoes, diced
1 cup minced parsley
4 green onions, chopped
½ cup minced fresh mint
  leaves
24 small romaine lettuce
  leaves

1. Soak the cracked wheat
in hot water to cover for
30 minutes. While the
cracked wheat is soaking,
make the dressing.

2. Combine the lemon juice
and salt and stir until the
salt is dissolved.

3. Add the pepper, garlic
and water and mix well,
then slowly add the oil,
stirring as you do. Put the
dressing in a jar with
a tightly fitting lid and
shake vigorously for
30 seconds. Set aside.

4. Drain the cracked wheat
thoroughly. Add the
tomatoes, parsley, green
onions and mint leaves to
the cracked wheat. Add
the dressing and toss
thoroughly. Chill well.

5. Serve on chilled salad
plates with each serving
surrounded by 4 romaine
leaves. Traditionally this
salad is eaten by scooping
it onto the romaine leaves
and eating out of hand.

Makes 8 servings
Each serving contains approximately:
  1 starch portion
  1 fat portion
  115 calories

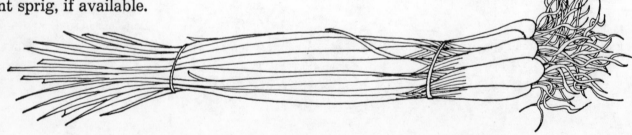

Simple Rice Salad

2¹/₂ cups Chicken Stock,
    page 30
1 cup long-grain white rice
³/₄ cup minced green onion
    tops
³/₄ cup minced parsley

1. Bring the stock to a boil
in a saucepan.

2. Add the rice, reduce
heat to low, cover and cook
for 25 minutes, or until all
of the liquid is absorbed
and the rice is fluffy.

3. Cool the rice to room
temperature, then refrigerate until cold.

4. Combine the rice, green
onion tops and parsley and
mix thoroughly.

Variations Add cold raw
or cooked vegetables of
choice. For an entree, add
cold cooked fish, poultry or
meat.

If you wish to serve this as
a hot salad, toss the hot
rice with the green onion
tops and parsley and serve
immediately.

Makes 10 servings (5 cups)
Each serving contains approximately:
    1 starch portion
    70 calories

Curried Tuna Salad

4 small heads Boston
    lettuce
1¹/₂ cups crushed pineapple
    canned in natural juice,
    undrained
Two 7-ounce cans water-
    packed tuna, drained and
    separated into bite-sized
    pieces
2 tablespoons raisins,
    finely chopped
¹/₂ cup Curried Yogurt
    Dressing, page 37

1. Remove the hearts from
the heads of lettuce, being
careful not to separate or
tear the outer leaves. Wash
the hearts, tear them into
bite-sized pieces (approximately 5 cups torn lettuce)
and put into a large bowl.
Retain the outer leaves for
lettuce "bowls" in which to
serve the salad. Wash the
"bowls" carefully and chill
until needed.

2. Add the pineapple and
its juice, the tuna, raisins
and dressing to the torn
lettuce and toss well.

3. Place each lettuce
"bowl" on a large chilled
plate and spoon an equal-
sized portion into each.

Makes 4 servings
Each serving contains approximately:
    2 low-fat protein portions
    1 fruit portion
    150 calories

Shrimp in Papaya Cups

2 ripe papayas
2 cups cooked shelled
    shrimp
¹/₄ cup minced chives or
    green onion tops
¹/₂ teaspoon curry powder
1 tablespoon sunflower
    seeds
4 parsley sprigs for garnish

1. Cut the papayas in half
lengthwise and carefully remove and discard the
seeds.

2. With a melon baller,
remove the papaya pulp
from the peel, being careful
not to tear the peel. Put
the balls in a mixing bowl
and set the peels aside.

3. Add the shrimp, chives
or green onion tops, curry
powder and sunflower
seeds to the melon balls
and mix well.

4. Divide the mixture
equally among the 4
reserved papaya halves.
Garnish each papaya cup
with a parsley sprig.

Makes 4 servings
Each serving contains approximately:
    1 fruit portion
    1/2 fat portion
    2 low-fat protein portions
    173 calories

Directions for Steaming Vegetables

When steaming vegetables, always make certain that the steamer basket is above the level of the water and that the water is boiling rapidly before the vegetables are covered and timing is begun.

Once the vegetables have steamed for the correct length of time, immediately place them under cold running water. This stops the cooking quickly and preserves both their color and texture.

When reheating vegetables prepared in this manner, be careful not to overcook them in the reheating process or they will lose both their crispness and their color.

Whether you are going to be serving vegetables hot or cold, they can be prepared in advance and stored, covered, in the refrigerator. Many of the recipes in this section call for steamed vegetables, and by being able to prepare them in advance, preparation at meal time can be greatly shortened.

In the following steaming chart, the time given for steaming each vegetable produces a crisp-tender result. Mushy, colorless vegetables are not only tasteless, but have been robbed of much of their nutritional value by overcooking.

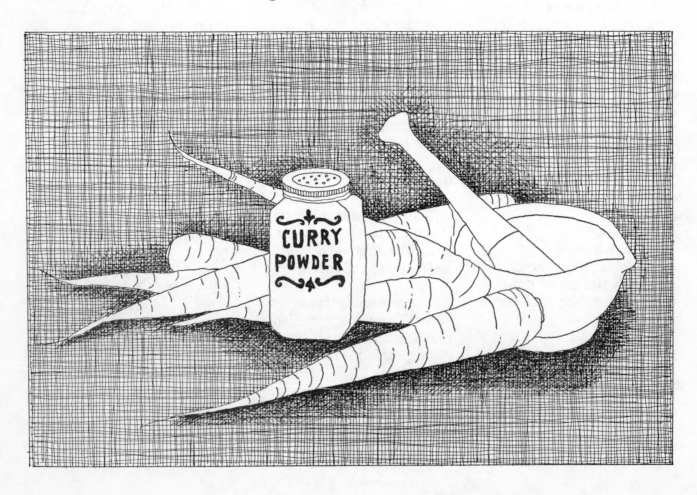

44

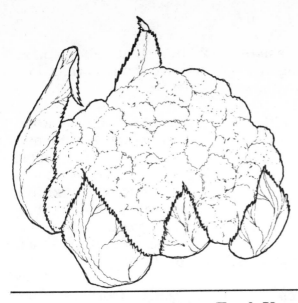

Fresh Vegetable Steaming Chart

Vegetable	Minutes	Vegetable	Minutes	Vegetable	Minutes
Asparagus	5	Corn		Pimientos	2
Beans:		kernels	3	Poke	3
green	5	on the cob	3	Potatoes:	
lima	5	Coriander (cilantro)	1–2	sweet, 1/2-inch slices	15
string or snap	5	Cucumber	2–3	white, 1/2-inch slices	10
Bean sprouts	1–2	Dandelion greens	1–2	Pumpkin	5
Beet greens	3–5	Eggplant	5	Radishes	5
Beets, quartered	15	Garlic	5	Rhubarb	5
Black radish, 1/2-inch slices	5	Jerusalem artichokes	8	Romaine lettuce	1–2
Breadfruit	10	Jicama	10	Rutabagas	8
Broccoli	5	Kale	1–2	Shallots	2
Brussels sprouts	5	Kohlrabi, quartered	8–10	Spinach	1–2
Cabbage, quartered	5	Leeks	5	Squash:	
Carrots, 1/2-inch slices	5	Lettuce	1–2	acorn	5
Cauliflower:		Lotus root, 1/4-inch slices	25	hubbard	5
flowerets	3	Mint	1–2	spaghetti	5
whole	5	Mushrooms	2	summer	3
Celery root	3–4	Mustard, fresh	1–2	zucchini	3
Celery stalks	10	Okra	5	Tomatoes	3
Chard	1–2	Onions:		Turnips, quartered	8
Chayote	3	green tops	3	Water chestnuts	8
Chicory	1–2	whole	5	Watercress	1–2
Chives	2–3	Palm hearts	5		
Collards	1–2	Parsley	1–2		
		Pea pods	3		
		Peas	3–5		
		Peppers:			
		chili	2–3		
		green and red bell	2		

Tomato Provençale

4 tomatoes
1/2 cup buttermilk
1/4 cup freshly grated Romano or Parmesan cheese
Salt
Freshly ground black pepper

1. Cut the tomatoes in half and remove the seeds. (If the tomatoes are very large, cut them in 1/2-inch slices.)

2. Drizzle 1 tablespoon of buttermilk into each tomato half.

3. Sprinkle the top of each tomato half with an equal amount of Romano or Parmesan cheese and season with salt and pepper.

4. Put the tomatoes in a 400° F oven for 15 minutes, then put them under the broiler until lightly browned.

Variations   Add a dash of oregano, basil, tarragon, garlic powder or rosemary to each tomato half.

Makes 8 servings
Each serving contains approximately:
    1 vegetable portion
    25 calories

Minted Peas

2 cups green peas (2 pounds unshelled)
1 teaspoon arrowroot
1/4 cup cold water
1 teaspoon fructose
4 teaspoons corn oil margarine
1/4 teaspoon salt
1/2 cup minced fresh mint leaves

1. Steam the peas until they are fork tender, about 2 minutes; be careful not to overcook them. Set aside and keep warm.

2. In a small saucepan, dissolve the arrowroot in the water.

3. Stir the fructose into the arrowroot mixture and place the pan over medium heat. Cook, stirring constantly, until the mixture comes to a boil. Continuing to stir, cook until the mixture is clear and thickened, about 2 minutes.

4. Remove from the heat and stir in the margarine and salt.

5. Pour the sauce over the steamed peas, add the mint and toss, mixing thoroughly.

Variation   Substitute sliced carrots for the peas.

Makes 8 servings
Each serving contains approximately:
    1 vegetable portion
    1/2 fat portion
    48 calories

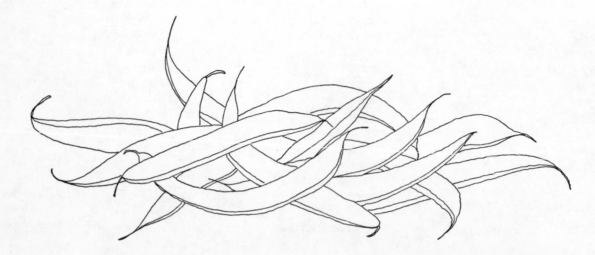

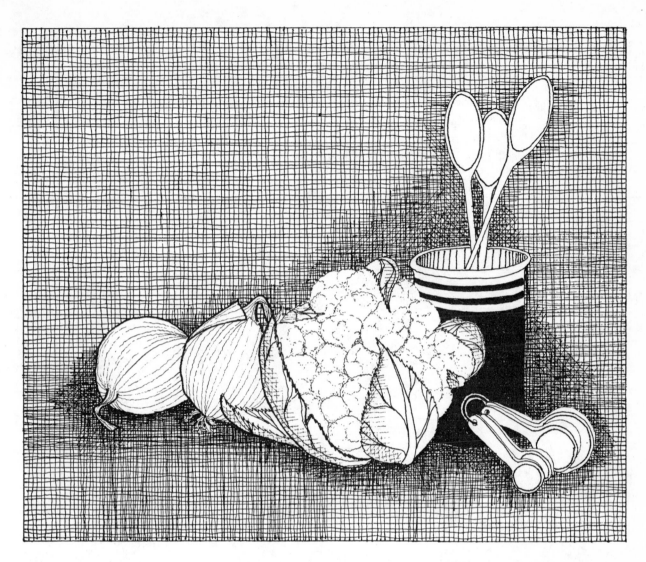

Cauliflower Incognito

1 large head cauliflower
1 tablespoon grated onion
1/4 teaspoon salt
1/8 teaspoon ground white
   pepper
1/8 teaspoon ground nutmeg

1. Preheat the oven to
350°F.

2. Break the cauliflower
into flowerets and cook in
very little water until fork
tender.

3. Drain the cauliflower,
reserving some of the cooking water, and mash it
with a little of the reserved
water.

4. Add all of the remaining
ingredients to the mashed
cauliflower and whip with
an electric mixer until
fluffy, or transfer to a
blender container and
blend until fluffy.

5. Transfer the mixture to
a casserole and bake in the
preheated oven for 20
minutes.

Makes 6 servings
Each serving contains approximately:
   1/2 vegetable portion
   13 calories

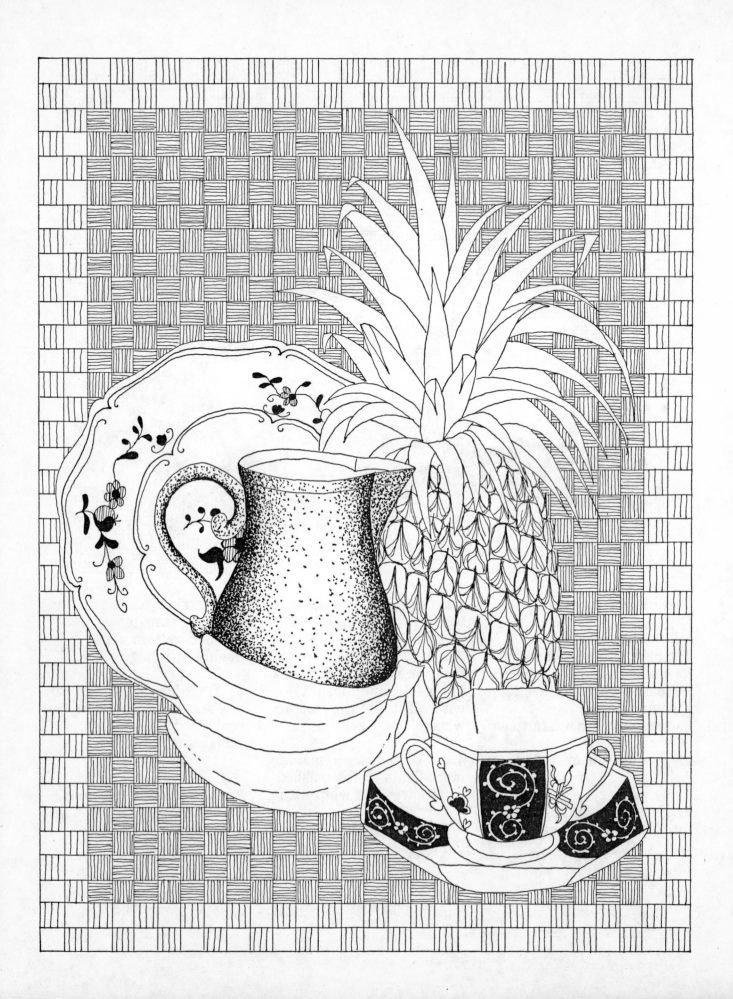

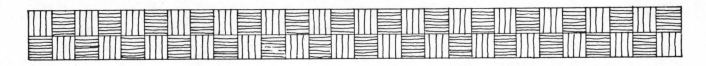

Eggs & Cheese

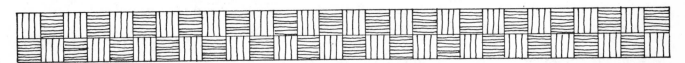

Soufflé Olé

2 tablespoons corn oil
   margarine
1/2 cup minced onion
1 large tomato, peeled and
   diced
1 1/2 teaspoons ground cumin
2 1/2 tablespoons flour
1 cup chicken stock, boiling
1/4 teaspoon salt
1/2 teaspoon chili powder
2 whole eggs, lightly beaten
1 cup grated Monterey
   Jack cheese
One 4-ounce can green chili
   peppers, seeded and
   chopped
6 egg whites, at room
   temperature
1/8 teaspoon cream of tartar
Dash of salt

1. Preheat the oven to
400°F. Melt the margarine
in a heavy saucepan large
enough to hold the entire
soufflé mixture prior to
putting it in the soufflé
dish.

2. Add the onion, tomato
and cumin and cook over
medium heat for 10 minutes, or until the onion is
tender and clear.

3. Add the flour, mix thoroughly and cook for 3 minutes, stirring constantly.
Do not brown.

4. Remove from the heat
and add the boiling stock
all at once, rapidly mixing
with a wire whisk to form
a smooth mixture.

5. Return the saucepan to
medium heat and simmer
for 3 to 4 minutes, stirring
frequently. When the mixture has thickened, remove
it from the heat and mix in
the salt and chili powder.

6. Slowly add the whole
eggs, stirring constantly.

7. Add the grated cheese
and chilies, mixing thoroughly.

8. Add the cream of tartar
and salt to the egg whites
and beat until stiff but
not dry.

9. Mix one fourth of the
egg whites into the soufflé
base to lighten it, then
gently fold in the remaining egg whites, being careful not to overmix.

10. Put the entire mixture into a soufflé dish
8 1/2 inches in diameter.
Place in the middle of the
preheated oven and cook
for 30 minutes.

11. Remove from the oven
and serve *immediately*.

Note Serve this soufflé
with hot corn tortillas and
a tossed green salad. If
there are leftovers, reheat
them and use as a vegetarian taco filling with
shredded lettuce, diced
tomatoes and a little taco
sauce.

Makes 6 servings
Each serving contains approximately:
   2 medium-fat protein portions
   150 calories

Soufflé Squares

4 eggs, separated
2 teaspoons butter or corn
  oil margarine, melted
1 cup (1/2 pint) low-fat
  small curd cottage cheese
1/4 cup whole-wheat pastry
  flour
1/4 teaspoon salt

1. Preheat the oven to
375°F.

2. Put the egg whites in a
clean, dry bowl. Put the
yolks in another large mixing bowl.

3. Beat the egg whites
until stiff but not dry.
Transfer the beater to the
yolks and beat until they
are light in color.

4. Beat the melted butter
or margarine, cottage
cheese, flour and salt into
the egg yolks.

5. Carefully fold the
beaten egg whites into the
yolk mixture.

6. Spoon the mixture into
a shallow 9- by 13-inch
baking dish that has been
sprayed with a nonstick
spray and spread evenly.

7. Bake uncovered in
the preheated oven for
20 minutes or until lightly
and evenly browned on
the top.

8. Remove from the oven
and cut into squares to
serve.

Makes 8 servings
Each serving contains approximately:
   1/2 medium-fat protein portion
   1/2 low-fat protein portion
   1/4 fat portion
   78 calories

Fondue Soufflé

4 slices white bread, crusts
  removed
1 cup grated Cheddar
  cheese (1/4 pound)
1/4 teaspoon Beau Monde
  seasoning
1/8 teaspoon ground white
  pepper
1/4 teaspoon dry mustard
1/4 teaspoon salt
4 eggs, lightly beaten
2 cups non-fat milk
2 tablespoons minced
  chives or green onion tops
1/4 teaspoon Worcestershire
  sauce

1. Set the bread on a
counter top and expose to
the air for several hours so
that it can be easily cubed.

2. Cut the bread into
1/4-inch squares and ar-

range half of the squares in
a single layer in a shallow
8- by 13-inch baking dish.

3. Sprinkle half of the
cheese evenly over the
bread. Repeat the layers,
using the remaining bread
cubes and cheese.

4. Add the Beau Monde
seasoning, white pepper,
mustard and salt to the
eggs and mix well. Add the
milk, mix thoroughly, and
then add the chives or
green onion tops and
Worcestershire sauce.

5. Pour the liquid mixture
over the cheese and bread
in the baking dish. Cover
and refrigerate overnight.

6. Two hours before cooking, remove the baking
dish from the refrigerator.
To cook, set the baking
dish in a shallow pan of
cold water and place in a
cold oven. Set the oven for
300°F and cook for 1 hour.
Check occasionally to make
sure the top is not getting
too brown. If necessary,
cover with aluminum foil
to prevent excessive
browning.

Makes 4 servings
Each serving contains approximately:
   1 starch portion
   2 medium-fat protein portions
   1/2 non-fat milk portion
   215 calories

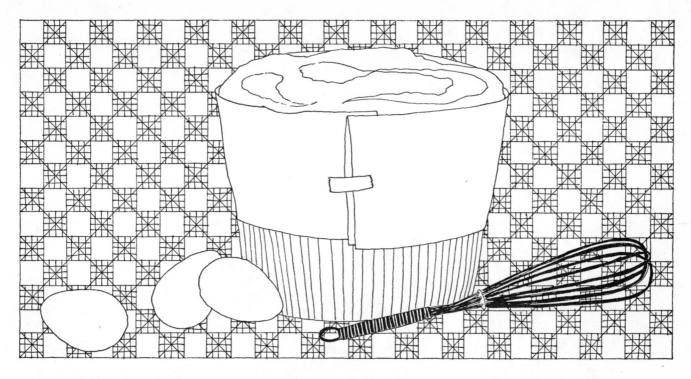

Poached Eggs

2 quarts water
2 tablespoons white
   vinegar
1 tablespoon fresh lemon
   juice
1 teaspoon salt
Eggs

1. Put the water, vinegar, lemon juice and salt in a large pan and bring to a boil.

2. When the water is boiling, break each egg in a saucer, one at a time, and quickly slide them into the water so that they will cook evenly.

3. Turn the heat down to simmer. Poach the eggs about 2 to 3 minutes, depending on how firm you want them. Do not put too many eggs in the pan at one time, as they are difficult to handle.

4. Remove the eggs from the water with a slotted spoon. Dip each egg into a bowlful of lightly salted warm water to rinse it. Then blot the eggs with paper toweling before serving.

Note Eggs may be poached a day ahead of serving and stored in the refrigerator. In order to store them, put them directly from the simmering water into a bowl filled with ice water. To reheat, put them in a large pan of warm water with a little salt and bring the water almost to a boil. Remove each egg with a slotted spoon, blot with paper toweling and serve.

Each egg contains approximately:
   1 medium-fat protein portion
   75 calories

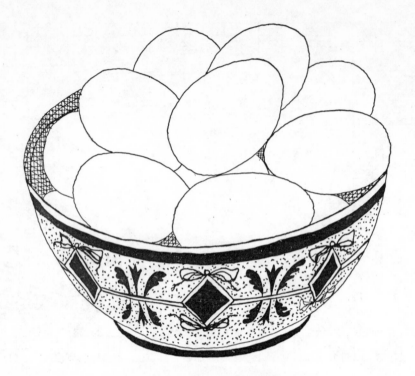

Eggs Foo Yung

Sauce
2 tablespoons soy sauce
2 teaspoons cornstarch
1 tablespoon cider vinegar
1/4 teaspoon salt
1/2 cup cold water
3/4 teaspoon fructose

Patties
1 cup bean sprouts,
   cooked and drained
1/2 cup minced green
   onion tops
1 cup chopped cooked
   shrimp
6 eggs, lightly beaten
2 teaspoons corn oil

1. To make the sauce, put the soy sauce, cornstarch, vinegar and salt in a saucepan and stir until smooth. Slowly stir in the water.

2. Cook over low heat, stirring constantly, until thickened. Mix in the fructose and set aside.

3. To make the patties, put the bean sprouts, green onion tops and shrimp in a bowl and mix well. Add the eggs and mix well.

4. Put the oil in a large cured heavy iron skillet and place over medium heat. When the skillet is hot, pour the egg mixture into the pan as if you are making pancakes, using about 1/4 cup for each patty.

5. When lightly browned on one side, turn over and brown the other side. Then turn the heat to low and continue cooking until the egg is completely done, about 5 minutes.

6. Reheat the sauce to serving temperature. Serve each patty with a little sauce spooned over it.

Makes 4 servings
Each serving contains approximately:
   2 medium-fat protein portions
   1/4 starch portion
   1/2 fat portion
   191 calories

Sourdough French Toast

4 eggs
1 cup buttermilk
1/8 teaspoon salt
4 slices sourdough French
   bread

1. The night before you wish to serve the French toast, combine the eggs, buttermilk and salt and mix well.

2. Place the slices of bread in a shallow glass baking dish and pour the egg mixture over the bread. Pierce the bread with the tines of a fork so that it will more rapidly absorb the egg mixture. Cover the dish and refrigerate overnight.

3. In the morning, remove the bread from the baking dish and place it on a baking sheet with a nonstick coating. Pour any egg mixture remaining in the baking dish over the bread.

4. Place the baking sheet under a preheated broiler until the bread is a golden brown in color, then turn the bread over and brown the other side.

Makes 4 servings
Each serving contains approximately:
   1 medium-fat protein portion
   1 starch portion
   1/4 non-fat milk portion
   165 calories

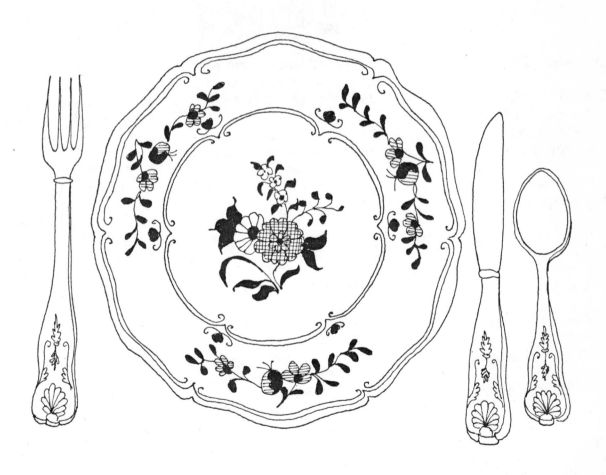

53

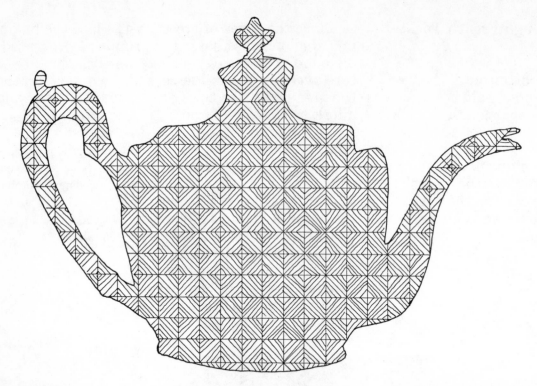

Breakfast Pizza

2 English muffins
1 cup (1/2 pint) low-fat cottage cheese
1 teaspoon ground cinnamon
1 teaspoon vanilla extract
1 tablespoon fructose

1. Cut the English muffins in half and, with a rolling pin, roll each half until it is well flattened.

2. Place the muffin halves under a preheated broiler until golden brown.

3. While the muffins are toasting, combine the cottage cheese, cinnamon, vanilla extract and fructose in a blender container and blend until smooth.

4. Spread each warm muffin half with 1/4 cup of the cottage-cheese mixture.

Makes 4 servings
Each serving contains approximately:
    1 starch portion
    1 low-fat protein portion
    1/4 fruit portion
135 calories

Carrots Indienne

1 tablespoon corn oil margarine
1 1/2 teaspoons curry powder
4 teaspoons grated ginger root, or 1 teaspoon ground ginger
8 medium carrots, grated
1/2 cup finely chopped chives
1/2 cup raisins
3 cups low-fat small curd cottage cheese

1. Melt the corn oil margarine in a skillet over medium heat, add the curry powder and ginger and mix thoroughly.

2. Add the carrots, chives and raisins and cook, stirring constantly, until just tender, about 10 minutes.

3. Add the cottage cheese, mix thoroughly and heat just to serving temperature. *Do not bring to a boil.*

Makes 8 servings
Each serving contains approximately:
    1 vegetable portion
    1/2 fruit portion
    1 1/2 low-fat protein portions
    1/4 fat portion
139 calories

Crêpes Florentine

2 cups partially skimmed
 ricotta cheese
4 cups chopped cooked
 spinach
1/2 cup finely chopped green
 onion tops
1/2 teaspoon garlic powder
1/4 teaspoon salt
2 tablespoons grated
 Romano cheese
8 Crêpes, page 73

1. Preheat the oven to
350°F.

2. Combine all of the ingredients, except the Romano cheese and crêpes, in a large mixing bowl and mix well.

3. Spoon one eighth of the mixture evenly down the center of each crêpe. Fold both sides of the crêpe over the filling toward the center and place, seam side down, in a glass baking dish. Repeat with remaining crêpes and filling.

4. Sprinkle the Romano cheese evenly over the tops of the crêpes.

5. Bake in the preheated oven for 20 minutes or until the cheese is lightly browned.

Makes 8 crêpes
Each crêpe contains approximately:
   1 medium-fat protein portion
   1/2 starch portion
   1 vegetable portion
   135 calories

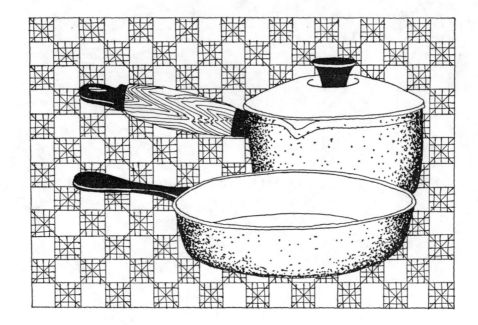

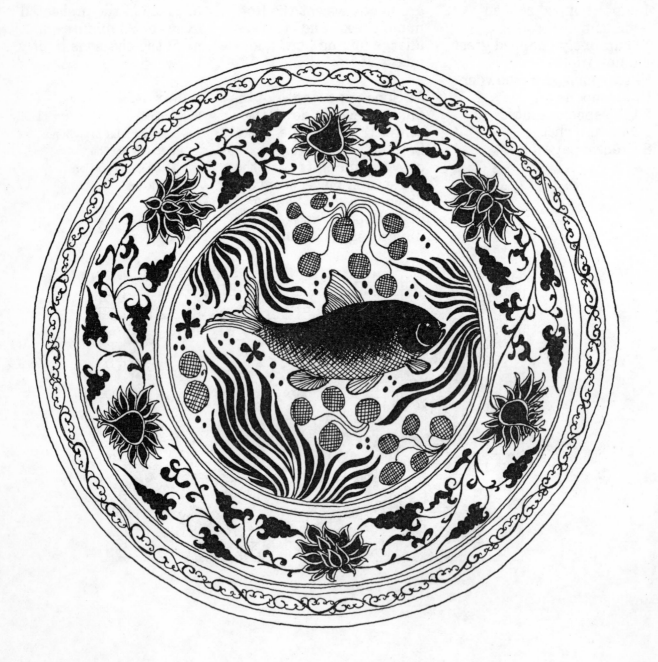

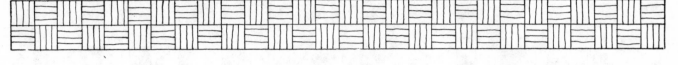

Seafood, Poultry & Meat

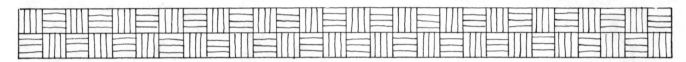

Seviche

1 pound snapper, cut into
  small cubes
Juice of 3 limes
Salt
Ground white pepper
Garlic salt
1 cup chopped onion
1/4 cup red-wine vinegar
2 teaspoons crumbled dried
  oregano
1/2 cup chopped fresh coriander (cilantro) or parsley
3 ripe tomatoes, peeled and
  chopped
One 4-ounce can jalapeño
  chili peppers, cut into
  strips, with the juice
  from the can
One 2-ounce can whole
  pimientos, cut into
  strips, with the juice
  from the can
1/2 cup Tomato Juice
  Catsup, page 27
Salt and freshly ground
  black pepper to taste

1. Place the cubed fish in a
glass dish and pour the
lime juice over it.

2. Lightly sprinkle the
salt, white pepper and
garlic salt over the fish.

3. Cover and refrigerate
for 24 hours.

4. Remove from the refrigerator and mix in all of the
remaining ingredients.

5. Cover and refrigerate
4 more hours before serving.

Makes 8 appetizer servings
Each serving contains approximately:
   2 low-fat protein portions
   1 vegetable portion
 135 calories

Eggplant in Clam Sauce

2 teaspoons corn oil
  margarine
Two 8-ounce cans chopped
  clams, drained and liquid
  reserved
2 cloves garlic, pressed
1 large eggplant, peeled
  and cut into 1/2-inch
  cubes
1/2 cup minced parsley
1/2 cup minced chives or
  green onion tops
1/4 cup freshly grated
  Parmesan cheese

1. Combine the margarine
and the liquid from the
clams in a cured heavy iron
skillet placed over low
heat.

2. Add the garlic and cook
slowly for a few minutes.

3. Add the eggplant and
cook over medium heat,
stirring from time to time,
for 15 minutes.

4. Add 1/4 cup of the
parsley and the chives
or green onions and cook
5 minutes.

5. Add the chopped clams,
Parmesan cheese and the
remaining 1/4 cup parsley.
Mix well and serve at once.
Further cooking will cause
the clams to toughen.

Makes 4 servings
Each serving contains approximately:
   1 low-fat protein portion
   1 vegetable portion
   1/2 fat portion
 103 calories

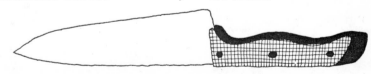

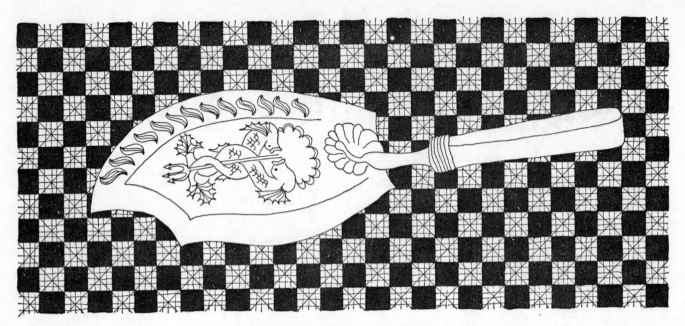

Fresh Fish Gumbo

Two 28-ounce cans solid-pack tomatoes, with the juice from the cans
1 large onion, chopped
3 cloves garlic, minced
1 green bell pepper, diced
3 sprigs parsley, chopped
1 quart water
1 teaspoon salt
1 teaspoon freshly ground black pepper
2 bay leaves
4 cups whole okra, steamed until tender and cut into pieces
Two 8-ounce cans tomato sauce
1½ pounds firm white fish, cubed

1. Heat a cured heavy iron skillet over medium heat and add ¼ cup of the juice from the tomatoes.

2. Add the onion, garlic, green pepper and parsley and cook until the onions are tender and clear.

3. Chop the tomatoes and put them in a large kettle with the remaining juice and the cooked onion mixture, cover and simmer 1 hour.

4. Add the water, salt, black pepper and bay leaves and simmer an additional hour.

5. Add the okra and tomato sauce and cook for 30 minutes.

6. Add the cubed fish and cook for 10 minutes.

Note If possible, make this dish up to the point where the fish is added the day before you plan to serve it. This allows time for the flavors to blend. Then reheat, add the fish and cook the final 10 minutes.

Makes 8 servings
Each serving contains approximately:
    2 low-fat protein portions
    2 vegetable portions
160 calories

58

Oysters Rockefeller

1 pound spinach, chopped
One 16-ounce jar shucked
   oysters, drained and
   liquor reserved
2 cups (1 recipe) Mornay
   Sauce, page 25
1 tablespoon grated
   Parmesan cheese
Paprika

1. Preheat the oven to
350°F.

2. Steam the spinach
until tender and drain
thoroughly, pressing out
all of the excess moisture;
set aside.

3. Place a skillet over
medium heat and add the
oysters with 2 tablespoons
of their liquor.

4. Cook the oysters
until they turn white and
the edges curl, about
5 minutes.

5. Line the bottom of a
shallow 8- by 12-inch
flameproof baking dish
with the reserved spinach,
arrange the oysters on top
and pour over the pan
juices.

6. Pour the Mornay Sauce
over the oysters, then
sprinkle with the Parmesan
cheese and a little paprika.

7. Bake in the preheated
oven for 10 minutes, then
lightly brown under the
broiler.

Makes 4 servings
Each serving contains approximately:
   1 1/2 low-fat protein portions
    3/4 fat portion
    1/2 non-fat milk portion
    1/4 starch portion
   172 calories

Red Snapper Veracruz

1 1/2 pounds snapper fillets
   (six 4-ounce fillets)
2 limes
1 teaspoon salt
1 teaspoon corn oil
1 cup sliced onion
One 4 1/2-ounce can whole
   pimientos
3 large ripe tomatoes,
   chopped
1 small fresh green chili
   pepper, seeded and
   chopped, or 1 teaspoon
   chopped canned green
   chili pepper
10 capers, chopped
1 sprig parsley

1. Rinse the fish fillets well
with cold water.

2. Squeeze the lime juice
on the fillets and rub them
with salt. Cover and refrigerate until ready to cook
(at least 2 hours).

3. Put the oil in a cured
heavy iron skillet and place
over medium heat. Add the
onion and cook until tender
and clear.

4. Drain the pimientos,
chop half of them and
reserve the other half for
garnish.

5. Add the chopped pi-
mientos, tomatoes, chili
pepper, capers and parsley
sprig to the onion and
cook, covered, until there
is juice to a depth of about
1 inch in the skillet.

6. Add the fillets and cook
for about 6 minutes on
each side, or until the fish
is completely white and
fork tender.

7. Transfer the fillets to a
serving platter and spoon
the sauce over the top,
discarding the parsley
sprig. Cut the remaining
pimientos into julienne
strips and garnish the
fillets.

Makes 8 servings
Each serving contains approximately:
   2 low-fat protein portions
   1/4 fat portion
   1/4 vegetable portion
   127 calories

59

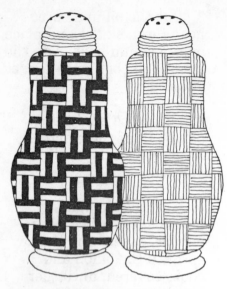

Italian Chicken

2 cups tomato juice
2 tablespoons red-wine
 vinegar
1/4 teaspoon salt
1 medium onion, thinly
 sliced
1 teaspoon crumbled dried
 oregano
1/4 teaspoon freshly ground
 black pepper
3 cups diced cooked
 chicken
1 cup grated mozzarella
 cheese

1. Put the tomato juice in
a large saucepan. Add the
vinegar, salt and onion and
mix thoroughly.

2. Bring the mixture to
a boil, reduce the heat and
simmer, uncovered, for
1 hour.

3. Add the oregano and
black pepper and continue
to simmer slowly, uncovered, for another 30 minutes.

4. Combine the tomato
sauce and chicken and mix
well.

5. Spread the tomato
sauce–chicken mixture in
the bottom of a flameproof
baking dish and sprinkle
the mozzarella cheese over
the top.

6. Place the dish under the
broiler until the cheese is
melted and lightly browned.

Makes 8 servings
Each serving contains approximately:
  3/4 vegetable portion
  1 1/2 low-fat protein portions
  1/2 medium-fat protein portion
  140 calories

Chicken Enchiladas

1 tablespoon corn oil
1 large onion, chopped
1 1/2 teaspoons salt
1 tablespoon chili powder
1/2 teaspoon ground cumin
2 medium tomatoes, peeled
 and diced
2 cups chopped cooked
 chicken
1/2 cup chicken stock
1 cup grated sharp
 Cheddar cheese
8 corn tortillas, warmed

1. Preheat the oven to
350°F.

2. Heat the corn oil in a
skillet, add the onion and
cook until tender and clear.

3. Add the salt, chili
powder and cumin and
mix well. Then mix in
the tomatoes, chicken and
chicken stock and cook for
5 minutes over low heat.

4. Remove from the heat,
add 3/4 cup of the cheese
and mix thoroughly.

5. Spoon an equal portion
of the chicken mixture
evenly down the center of
each warm tortilla. Fold
the sides over the filling so
that they overlap and place
seam side down in a lightly
greased baking dish. Spoon
any remaining sauce evenly
over the enchiladas and
then sprinkle the remaining 1/4 cup of cheese over
the top.

6. Cover the baking dish
and bake in the preheated
oven for 30 minutes.

Makes 8 servings
Each serving contains approximately:
  1/4 fat portion
  1/4 vegetable portion
  1 starch portion
  1 low-fat protein portion
  1 high-fat protein portion
  237 calories

Chinese Chicken with Snow Peas

3 whole chicken breasts, poached until tender
2 teaspoons Oriental-style sesame oil
1/2 pound bean sprouts
1/2 pound Chinese snow peas (pea pods)
1 cup chopped green onions
2 cups sliced fresh mushrooms (1/2 pound)
1 cup Chicken Stock, page 30
2 tablespoons soy sauce
1 teaspoon grated ginger root
1/2 teaspoon salt
1 teaspoon fructose
1 1/2 tablespoons cornstarch
2 tablespoons cold water

1. Remove the skin, fat and bones from the chicken breasts. Cut the meat into 1/2-inch-wide strips. Set aside.

2. Heat the oil in a skillet over medium heat and add the bean sprouts, snow peas, green onions and mushrooms. Cook, stirring, a few minutes until the vegetables are just tender.

3. Add the stock, soy sauce, ginger root, salt and fructose and mix well. Cover and cook 2 minutes.

4. Dissolve the cornstarch in the cold water and add to the pan. Cook, stirring, until the pan liquids are clear and slightly thickened.

5. Add the chicken strips, mix well and heat through. Serve with white rice.

Makes 8 servings
Each serving contains approximately:
2 low-fat protein portions
1/4 fat portion
1 vegetable portion
146 calories
1/2 cup cooked white rice contains approximately:
1 starch portion
70 calories

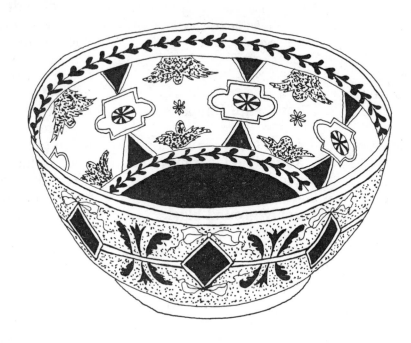

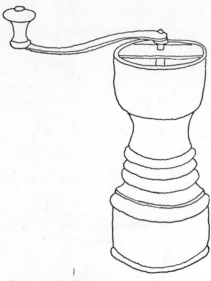

Shish Kebabs

1 pound lean lamb, cut into
 1-inch cubes
12 cherry tomatoes
1 green bell pepper, cut
 into 1-inch squares
12 small boiling onions,
 parboiled 3 minutes

Marinade
1/2 cup red-wine vinegar
2 tablespoons soy sauce
1/4 teaspoon freshly ground
 black pepper
Dash cayenne pepper
1 teaspoon salt
1/2 cup minced onion
1 tablespoon crumbled
 dried oregano

1. Combine all of the in-
gredients for the marinade.

2. Put the lamb cubes in a
glass or ceramic dish and
pour the marinade over
them. Cover and marinate,
refrigerated, 8 hours.

3. Remove the lamb cubes
from the marinade, reserving the marinade. Thread
the lamb cubes on skewers
alternately with the
tomatoes, green pepper
squares and onions. Put
the skewers back in the
marinade for 1 to 2 hours.

4. Broil the shish kebabs
in a preheated broiler or
grill over a charcoal fire
until the lamb is cooked
as desired.

Makes 6 servings
Each serving contains approximately:
   2 low-fat protein portions
   1 vegetable portion
 135 calories

Dijon Lamb Chops

4 small thick lamb chops,
 all visible fat removed
1 lemon
Garlic salt
Freshly ground black
 pepper
1/3 cup Dijon-style mustard
4 teaspoons unprocessed
 wheat bran
1 cup finely chopped parsley

1. Preheat the oven to
500°F.

2. Place the lamb chops in
a shallow baking dish and
rub both sides of each chop
with lemon. Then sprinkle
both sides of each with garlic salt and black pepper.

3. Combine the mustard,
bran and parsley and mix
well. Cover each lamb chop
with an equal amount of
the parsley mixture, pressing it down firmly with
your hands.

5. Put the lamb chops in
the preheated oven for
4 minutes. Then turn the
oven *off* and *do not open*
the door for 30 minutes.

Note This is an ideal dinner entree for busy people
who give dinner parties.
You can prepare the lamb
chops many hours in ad-
vance or even a day ahead
of time. Cover them tightly
and refrigerate until you
are 34 minutes from serv-
ing time. (Even if you
leave them in a little
longer than 30 minutes
after the oven is turned off
the chops will not be over-
cooked.) If you prefer lamb
chops well done, bake them
for 5 minutes instead of 4
before turning off the oven.

Makes 4 servings
Each serving contains approximately:
   2 low-fat protein portions
 110 calories

Dieter's Spicy Sausage

2 pounds lean ground pork (*absolutely* all visible fat removed before grinding)
2 teaspoons ground sage
1 teaspoon freshly ground black pepper
1 teaspoon fructose
3/4 teaspoon garlic powder
1/2 teaspoon onion powder
1/2 teaspoon ground mace
1/4 teaspoon ground allspice
1/4 teaspoon salt
1/8 teaspoon ground cloves

1. Combine all of the ingredients in a large mixing bowl and mix thoroughly.

2. Form into 12 patties and cook over medium heat in a nonstick pan until lightly browned on both sides.

Note This recipe may be doubled and the extra patties frozen in individual plastic bags. Also, the flavor improves if made a day before you plan to cook them. These patties are not only much lower in calories than any other sausage, but they are also more delicious.

Makes 12 patties
Each patty contains approximately:
    2 medium-fat protein portions
    150 calories

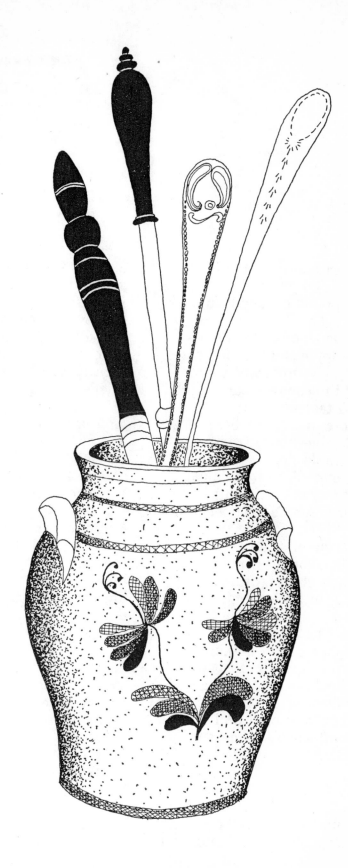

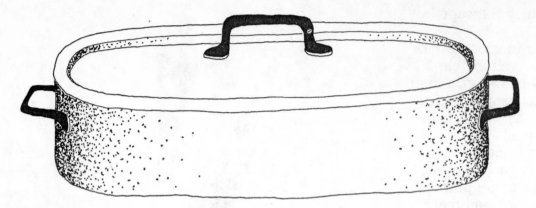

Cantonese Pork

1 pound cooked lean pork
  roast
One 20-ounce can pine-
  apple chunks in natural
  juice, undrained
2 tablespoons cornstarch
1/2 teaspoon salt
1/3 cup cider vinegar
3 tablespoons fructose
1 tablespoon soy sauce
1 cup sliced fresh mush-
  rooms (1/4 pound)
1/2 green bell pepper, thinly
  sliced
1/2 onion, thinly sliced
One 6-ounce can water
  chestnuts, drained and
  thinly sliced

1. Cut the roast pork in
1-inch cubes, making sure
to remove all fat. (You
should have 4 cups of
cubed meat. It is easiest to
remove the fat and cut the
pork when the meat is
cold.)

2. Drain the juice from the
pineapple chunks, set the
chunks aside and pour the
juice into a large saucepan.

3. Add the cornstarch,
salt and vinegar to the
juice, stirring well to
dissolve the cornstarch and
salt. Place over medium
heat and cook, stirring constantly, until the sauce has
thickened.

4. Remove from the heat
and add the fructose, soy
sauce, pineapple chunks
and pork. Let the mixture
stand for 1 hour.

5. Return the pan to the
heat and add the mush-
rooms, bell pepper, onion
and water chestnuts. Cook
until the vegetables are
done, but still slightly
crisp. Serve with white
rice.

Makes 8 servings
Each serving contains approximately:
    2 low-fat protein portions
    1 fruit portion
    1/2 vegetable portion
    163 calories
1/2 cup cooked white rice contains
approximately:
    1 starch portion
    70 calories

Popeye's Hash

1 pound spinach, chopped
1 pound ground lean beef
1 cup chopped onion
2 eggs, lightly beaten
1/2 teaspoon salt

1. Steam the spinach until
tender and drain thor-
oughly, pressing out all of
the excess moisture; set
aside.

2. Put the ground beef and
onion in a cured heavy iron
skillet and sauté over
medium heat until the
meat is cooked and the
onion is tender and clear.

3. Add the chopped
spinach to the meat mix-
ture and mix well.

4. Add the eggs and salt
to the skillet and cook,
stirring, until the egg is
completely set.

Makes 4 servings
Each serving contains approximately:
    3 medium-fat protein portions
    1 vegetable portion
    250 calories

Steak au Poivre

One 3-pound top sirloin
steak, 1¼ inches thick
2 tablespoons black
peppercorns
1 teaspoon corn oil
margarine
½ cup dry white wine
1 tablespoon brandy

1. Begin preparing the
steak 2 hours before you
wish to serve it. Remove
all of the visible fat, wipe
with a damp cloth and
carefully dry it.

2. Crush the peppercorns
in a mortar with a pestle
or put them in a cloth and
pound them with a ham-
mer. (This amount of pep-
percorns will result in a
very "hot" pepper steak.
For a milder flavor, use
only 1 to 2 teaspoons.)

3. Press the crushed pep-
percorns firmly into both
sides of the steak with
your hands. Then "smack"
the steak all over with the
flat side of a meat cleaver
to press the pepper in more
securely. Cover the steak
and allow it to stand at
room temperature until
you are ready to cook it.

4. In a large, cured iron
skillet, melt the margarine,
then wipe it out with paper
toweling. Place the skillet
over high heat until very
hot, then put the steak in
it and cook for 5 minutes
on each side (for rare).

5. Remove the steak to a
heated platter and pour the
white wine and brandy into
the skillet. Allow to boil
for 2 minutes, stirring constantly and scraping all
the drippings from the bottom of the skillet into the
wine.

6. Remove the pan from
the heat and pour the con-
tents into a heated sauce
dish or gravy boat.

7. Slice the steak horizontally into very thin slices.
Spoon a little of the sauce
over each serving.

Each slice (1 by 3 by ¼ inch)
contains approximately:
   1 low-fat protein portion
   55 calories

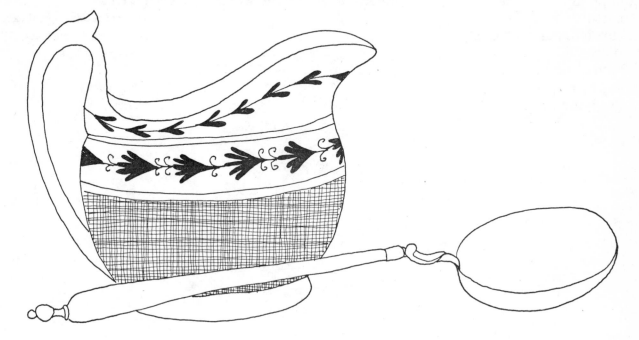

65

Jones Stew

1½ pounds boned lean
  beef, cut into 1-inch cubes
½ cup all-purpose flour
4 teaspoons corn oil
  margarine
2 leeks, white part only,
  thinly sliced
2 cups sliced fresh mush-
  rooms (½ pound)
2 sprigs parsley, minced
1 clove garlic, pressed
1 bay leaf
½ teaspoon crumbled dried
  thyme
½ teaspoon crumbled dill
  weed
½ teaspoon crumbled dried
  summer savory
1 teaspoon salt
½ teaspoon freshly ground
  black pepper
1½ cups water
2 cups dry red wine
1 carrot, sliced
2 turnips, cut into large
  pieces
10 small boiling onions
2 cups green peas
  (2 pounds unshelled)

1. Put the cubed beef and flour in a paper bag and shake until the meat is thoroughly coated.

2. Melt the margarine in the bottom of a heavy soup kettle over medium heat and add the leeks and mushrooms. Saute until tender; remove from the pan and set aside. Do not wash the pan.

3. Add the meat to the hot pan and, over medium-high heat, brown rapidly. When the meat is brown, return the leeks and mushrooms to the pan.

4. Add the parsley, garlic, bay leaf, thyme, dill weed, summer savory, salt, black pepper, ½ cup of the water and 1 cup of the wine, cover and simmer for 1 hour.

5. Add the remaining 1 cup of water and 1 cup of wine and simmer, covered, for 30 minutes.

6. Remove from the heat, cool and refrigerate over-night.

7. Lift all fat from the top and discard. Reheating slowly, bring to a boil and add all the vegetables, except the peas.

8. Simmer, covered, for 1 hour. Add the peas and cook until they are tender, 6 to 8 minutes.

Makes 8 servings
Each serving contains approximately:
  2 low-fat protein portions
  1 vegetable portion
  ½ fat portion
  ¼ starch portion
  176 calories

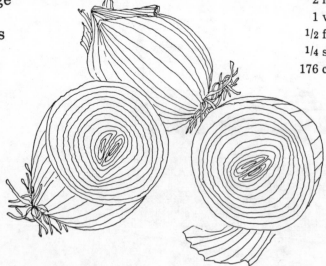

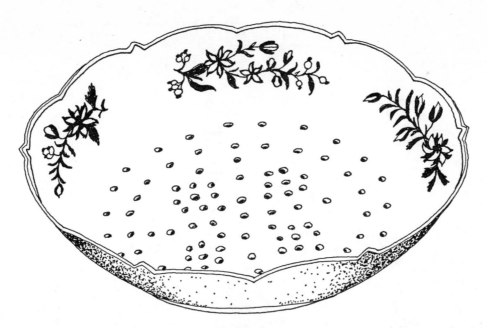

Rapid Roast

One 6-pound boneless beef
  roast
1 clove garlic
Salt

1. Preheat the oven to
500°F.

2. Rub the roast with the
garlic clove and salt it
generously. Put it in a
roasting pan in the pre-
heated oven for 30 min-
utes, then turn the
heat off.

3. Do not open the oven
door for exactly 2 hours,
then open it and remove
the roast. Let the roast
stand 15 minutes before
carving.

Note To serve the roast
au jus, use Beef Stock,
page 29, or Defatted Drippings, page 21, from your
freezer. Because so little of
the juice is lost in this
method of cooking, you
will find the drippings are
almost 100 percent fat.

Leaving the oven on for
30 minutes will result in a
rare roast. If you wish
well-done meat, cook it for
33 or 34 minutes at 500°F
before turning the heat off.
The general rule is: 5 minutes to the pound for rare
meat and 5 1/2 to 6 minutes
to the pound for well-done
meat.

Each slice (3 by 2 by 1/8 inch)
contains approximately:
   1 low-fat protein portion
   55 calories

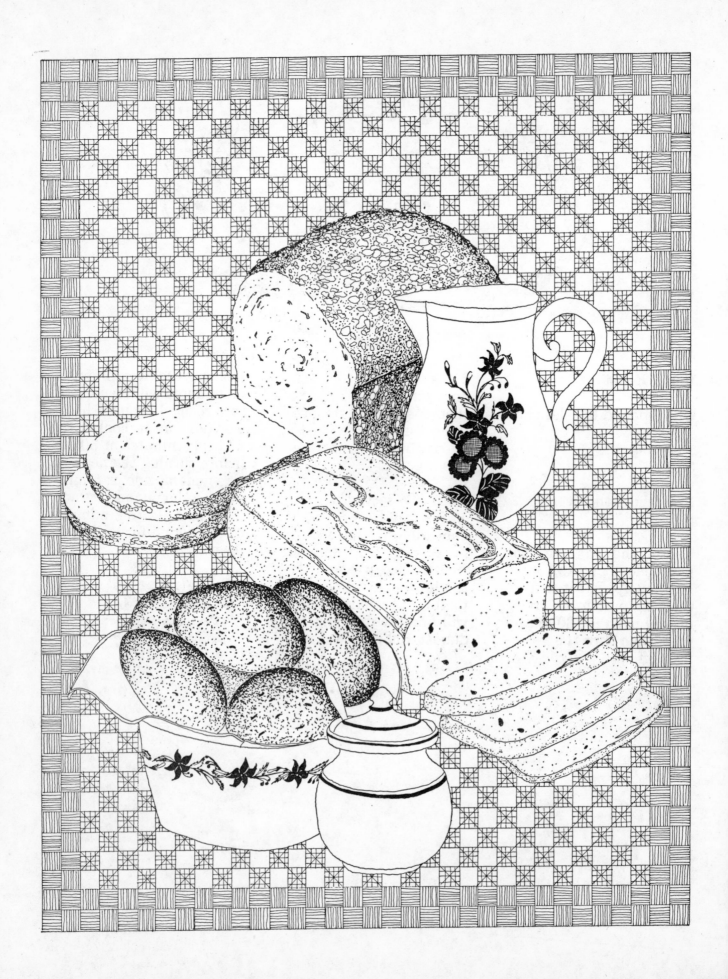

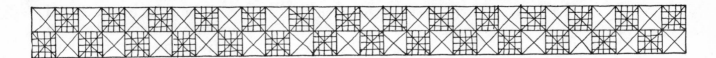

Breads & Cereals

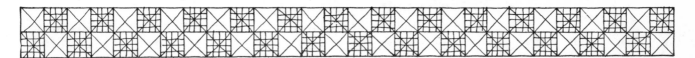

Canyon Ranch Bread

1¼ cups non-fat milk
1 tablespoon fresh lemon
  juice
¼ cup finely chopped
  raisins
1 cup unprocessed wheat
  bran
¼ cup liquid fructose
1 tablespoon vanilla extract
1 egg, lightly beaten, or
  ¼ cup liquid egg sub-
  stitute
1½ cups whole-wheat flour
1 tablespoon low-sodium
  baking powder, page 19

1. Combine the milk and
lemon juice in a large mixing bowl and mix well. Let
stand for 5 minutes.

2. Add the raisins, wheat
bran, liquid fructose and
vanilla extract to the bowl
and mix well. Cover and let
stand for 30 minutes.

3. Preheat the oven to
350°F.

4. Mix the egg or egg
substitute into the bran
mixture.

5. Combine the whole-
wheat flour and low-sodium
baking powder in a large
bowl and mix well. Add
the liquid ingredients to
the dry ingredients and
blend thoroughly.

6. Spray a standard-sized
metal loaf pan with a
nonstick spray. Transfer
the batter to the pan and
bake in the preheated oven
for 1 hour, or until a
wooden pick inserted in the
center comes out clean.

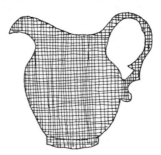

Remove the bread from the
oven and place it on its
side on a rack to cool.

7. When the bread is cool
enough to handle, remove
it from the pan and cool on
the rack to room tempera-
ture. Wrap the cooled
bread tightly in aluminum
foil and refrigerate until
cold before slicing.

8. To serve, slice the loaf
in half lengthwise, then cut
each half into 12 slices.
Light spread each slice
with corn oil margarine, if
desired. Rewrap the bread
in foil and reheat in a preheated 325°F oven for
30 minutes.

Makes 1 loaf; 24 slices
Each slice contains approximately:
  ¼ fruit portion
  ½ starch portion
  45 calories

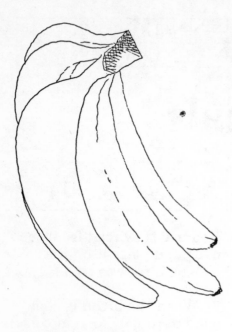

Banana Bread

2 cups all-purpose flour
1/8 teaspoon salt
1 1/2 teaspoons baking soda
2/3 cup fructose
6 tablespoons corn oil
    margarine, at room
    temperature
2 eggs, lightly beaten
1/2 cup buttermilk
1 teaspoon vanilla extract
3 ripe bananas, peeled and
    mashed

1. Preheat the oven to 350°F.

2. Combine 1 cup of the flour, the salt, baking soda and fructose in a large mixing bowl.

3. Add the margarine to the flour mixture and cream until smooth.

4. Add the beaten eggs and mix well.

5. Add the remaining 1 cup of flour alternately with the buttermilk, mixing well after each addition.

6. Add the vanilla extract and bananas and mix well.

7. Lightly grease and flour a standard-sized metal loaf pan and transfer the batter into it. Bake in the preheated oven for 1 hour, or until a wooden pick inserted in the center comes out clean. Remove the bread from the oven and place it on its side on a rack to cool.

8. When the bread is cool enough to handle, remove it from the pan and cool on the rack to room temperature. Wrap the cooled bread tightly in foil and refrigerate until cold before slicing.

9. To serve, slice the loaf thinly, wrap tightly in foil and put in a 300°F oven for about 10 minutes, or until it is hot.

Makes 1 loaf; 18 slices
Each slice contains approximately:
    1 starch portion
    1 fat portion
    1 fruit portion
155 calories

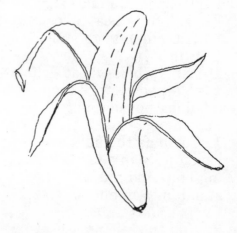

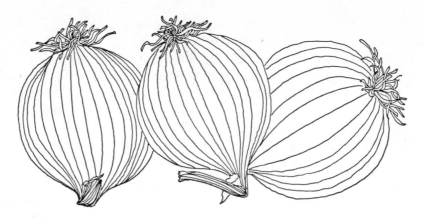

Dilled Onion Bread

1 yeast cake, or 1 envelope
(1 tablespoon) active dry
yeast
$1/4$ cup warm water
1 cup ($1/2$ pint) low-fat small
curd cottage cheese
4 teaspoons fructose
$1/4$ cup minced onion
$1/4$ teaspoon baking soda
1 egg, lightly beaten
2 tablespoons dill seed
1 teaspoon salt
2 cups all-purpose flour

1. Soften the yeast in the
warm water and let stand
for a few minutes.

2. Heat the cottage cheese
in a saucepan placed over
low heat and add the
dissolved yeast. Remove
from the heat.

3. Add the fructose, onion,
baking soda, egg, dill seed
and salt to the cottage
cheese mixture and mix
well.

4. Add the flour, a little at
a time, mixing well. Form
into a ball, cover and let
stand at room temperature
for several hours, or until
doubled in bulk.

5. Stir the dough until
again reduced to original
size, form into a loaf shape
and transfer to a well-oiled,
standard-sized metal loaf
pan. Cover the loaf pan
and allow the dough to
again double in bulk.

6. Preheat the oven to
350°F.

7. Bake the bread in the
preheated oven for 40 minutes, or until it makes a
hollow sound when tapped.

Note This bread is
delicious right from the
oven. It is much easier to
slice, however, when cool.
Wrap the sliced bread in
aluminum foil and store in
the refrigerator until ready
to use, then warm in the
foil in a 300°F oven before
serving.

Makes 1 loaf; 18 slices
Each slice contains approximately:
   1 starch portion
   70 calories

71

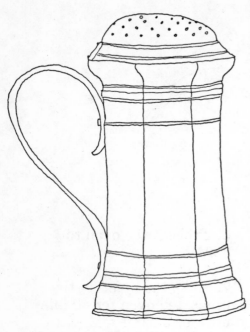

Toasted Tortilla Triangles

12 corn tortillas
Salt

1. Preheat the oven to 400°F.

2. Cut each tortilla into 6 pie wedge-shaped pieces.

3. Spread out half of the tortilla triangles on a baking sheet and salt lightly.

4. Place the baking sheet in the preheated oven for 10 minutes.

5. Remove the sheet from the oven, turn each triangle over and return to the oven for 3 more minutes.

6. Remove the baking sheet from the oven and transfer the tortilla triangles to a flat surface to cool.

7. Place the second half of the tortilla triangles on the baking sheet and repeat the process.

Note If you prefer smaller chips, cut the tortillas into smaller triangles before toasting them.

Makes 72 triangles
6 tortilla triangles contain approximately:
    1 starch portion
    70 calories

Cinnamon Popovers

4 egg whites, at room temperature
1 cup non-fat milk, at room temperature
1 cup all-purpose flour
2 tablespoons unsalted butter or corn oil margarine, melted
1/4 teaspoon fructose
1/2 teaspoon ground cinnamon

1. Preheat the oven to 450°F.

2. Put all of the ingredients in a blender container and blend at medium speed for 15 seconds. *Do not overmix.*

3. Divide the batter evenly among eight 4-ounce custard cups that have been well sprayed with a non-stick coating. (Only non-stick spray will prevent the popovers from sticking; butter or margarine won't do the job.)

4. Bake in the preheated oven for 20 minutes. Reduce the heat to 350°F and bake for 20 additional minutes.

Note The popovers may be frozen and reheated.

Makes 8 popovers
Each popover contains approximately:
    1 starch portion
    3/4 fat portion
    104 calories

Crêpes

1 cup non-fat milk
3/4 cup all-purpose flour
1/4 teaspoon salt
2 eggs, lightly beaten, or
  1/2 cup liquid egg sub-
  stitute
1 teaspoon corn oil mar-
  garine

1. Put the milk, flour and salt in a bowl and beat with an egg beater until well mixed.

2. Add the eggs or egg substitute and mix well.

3. In a 7-inch omelet or crêpe pan, melt the margarine over medium heat. When the margarine is melted and the pan is hot, tilt the pan to make sure the entire inner surface is coated.

4. Pour the melted margarine from the pan into the crêpe batter and mix well. Pour in just enough batter to barely cover the bottom of the pan (about 2 tablespoons) and tilt the pan from side to side to spread the batter evenly.

5. Place the pan on the heat, and when the edges of the crêpe start to curl, carefully turn the crêpe with a spatula and brown the other side.

6. Slide the crêpe from the pan and repeat with the remaining batter. To keep the crêpes pliable, put them in a covered casserole in a warm oven as you make them.

Makes 12 crêpes
Each crêpe contains approximately:
  1/2 starch portion
  35 calories

Powerful Porridge

1 cup unprocessed wheat
  bran
1 1/2 cups rolled oats
1/4 cup chopped almonds
3/4 cup chopped dried
  prunes
1/2 cup raisins
1 teaspoon ground
  cinnamon
3 cups water

1. Combine all of the dry ingredients in a mixing bowl and mix well.

2. Add the water, mix well, cover and refrigerate overnight. If possible, wait 2 or 3 days before serving. Serve cold.

Makes 4 cups
1/2 cup contains approximately:
  1 starch portion
  1/4 fat portion
  1 1/4 fruit portions
  131 calories

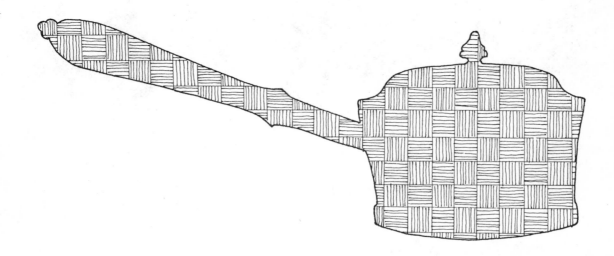

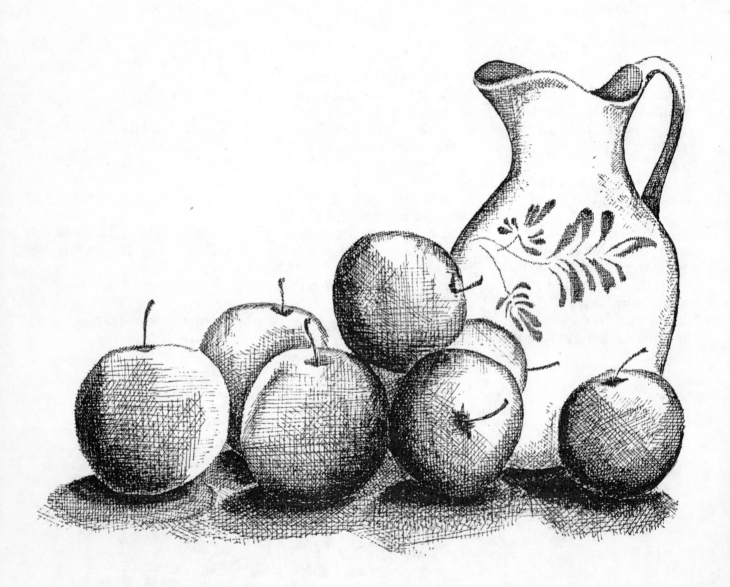

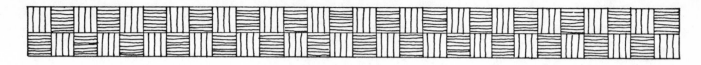

Desserts

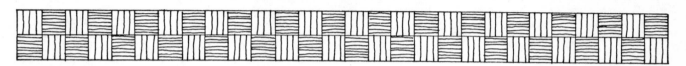

Sabino Spoof with Whoopee Topping

1 envelope (1 tablespoon)
   unflavored gelatin
1¼ cups cold water
¾ cup water, boiling
2 tablespoons fructose
¼ teaspoon vanilla extract
1 teaspoon rum extract
1 cup Whoopee Topping,
   following
Fresh mint sprigs

1. Put the gelatin in a small bowl, add ¼ cup of the cold water and let stand for 5 minutes.

2. Add the boiling water and stir until the gelatin is completely dissolved.

3. Stir in the fructose and extracts and refrigerate until firm.

4. When the mixture is firm, transfer to a blender container, add the remaining cup of cold water and blend until frothy.

5. Pour into sherbet glasses, add a dollop of Whoopee Topping to each serving and garnish with mint sprigs.

Makes 8 servings
Each serving contains approximately:
   ¼ fruit portion
   10 calories

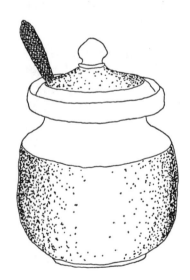

Whoopee Topping

1 cup canned skim milk,
   chilled
1 teaspoon vanilla extract
2 tablespoons fructose

1. Chill a mixing bowl and a rotary beater or beaters for an electric mixer in the freezer.

2. When ready to prepare, combine all of the ingredients in the chilled bowl and whip with the chilled beaters until the mixture is the desired consistency. Serve *immediately*.

Makes 5 scant cups
2 tablespoons contain approximately:
Free food
Calories negligible

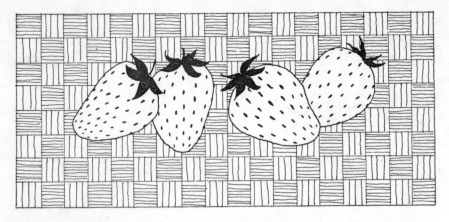

Strawberries Hoffmann-La Roche

1 cup non-fat milk
1 tablespoon cornstarch
2 tablespoons fructose
1 1/2 teaspoons vanilla
  extract
2 tablespoons Grand
  Marnier
2 egg whites, at room
  temperature
1/8 teaspoon cream of tartar
4 cups sliced fresh strawberries
8 whole strawberries

1. Put the milk in a saucepan. Add the cornstarch
and fructose and stir until
the cornstarch is thor-
oughly dissolved.

2. Place the pan on low
heat and bring to a boil.
Simmer, stirring constantly
with a wire whisk, until
slightly thickened.

3. Remove from the heat
and cool to room tempera-
ture.

4. Add the vanilla extract
and Grand Marnier to the
cooled sauce and mix well.

5. Combine the egg whites
and cream of tartar in a
bowl and beat until stiff
but not dry.

6. Fold the beaten egg
whites into the sauce, then
combine the sauce and the
sliced strawberries and
mix well.

7. Divide the mixture
evenly among 8 sherbet
glasses. Place a whole
strawberry on top of each
serving.

Makes 8 servings
Each serving contains approximately:
    1 starch portion
    70 calories

Tropical Fruit Cup

1 cup (1/2 pint) plain low-
  fat yogurt
1 ripe banana, sliced
1 orange, peeled and diced
  (a large navel orange is
  best)
1 cup diced fresh pineapple
  or unsweetened canned
  pineapple chunks cut in
  half
Ground cinnamon
Fresh mint sprigs

1. Put the yogurt and
banana in a blender con-
tainer and blend until
smooth.

2. Combine the orange and
pineapple in a mixing bowl
and pour the banana-
yogurt sauce over them.

3. Mix well and divide
evenly among 6 glasses.

4. Garnish with cinnamon
and mint sprigs.

Makes 6 servings
Each serving contains approximately:
    1 fruit portion
    40 calories

Citrus Compote

3 oranges
1/2 cup water
1/2 teaspoon vanilla extract
1/8 teaspoon ground cloves
2 teaspoons fructose

1. Grate enough orange peel to measure 1 tablespoon. Be careful to use only the orange-colored part and none of the white membrane. Set aside.

2. Peel the oranges and dice them over a bowl to catch the juice. Set the diced oranges aside.

3. Pour the juice into a saucepan and add the grated orange peel, water, vanilla extract and ground cloves.

4. Bring to a boil and boil for 3 minutes. Add the diced oranges and simmer for 10 minutes.

5. Cool and refrigerate. When cold, add the fructose and mix well.

Note This is excellent served chilled as a light dessert. It is also good as an omelet filling, as a sauce for French toast and pancakes, or, when warmed, as sauce for broiled chicken.

Makes 4 servings
Each serving contains approximately:
    1 fruit portion
    40 calories

Baked Apples

6 small green cooking apples
2 cups water
2 teaspoons vanilla extract
1/2 teaspoon ground cinnamon
1/2 cup fructose

1. Preheat the oven to 350°F.

2. Wash and core the apples. Remove the peel from the top third of each apple.

3. Arrange the apples in a baking dish just large enough to hold them snugly.

4. In a saucepan, bring the water, vanilla extract, cinnamon and fructose to a boil and pour over the apples.

5. Bake the apples in the preheated oven for 1 hour, or until they can be easily pierced with a fork. Baste the apples frequently as they cook.

6. When the apples are done, remove them from the oven and let cool in the sauce.

Note These apples are good served hot or cold. Try them with Whoopee Topping, sprinkled with cinnamon.

Makes 6 servings
Each serving contains approximately:
    2 fruit portions
    80 calories

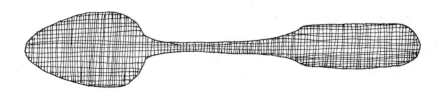

77

Melon Ball Compote

2/3 cup unsweetened apple
  juice
2 teaspoons arrowroot
1/2 teaspoon ground anise
  seed
1 teaspoon fructose
4 cups cantaloupe balls
  (2 medium-sized canta-
  loupes)

1. Combine the apple juice
and arrowroot in a sauce-
pan and stir until the arrowroot is completely
dissolved.

2. Add the anise seed and
fructose and mix thor-
oughly.

3. Slowly bring the mix-
ture to a boil and simmer
until slightly thickened,
stirring frequently.

4. Remove the pan from
the heat and cool to room
temperature.

5. Combine the sauce with
the melon balls and chill
before serving.

Note This is an unusual
and delicious dessert. It
also may be served as an
appetizer or may be com-
bined with cottage cheese
for a luncheon salad.

Makes 8 servings
Each serving contains approximately:
  1 fruit portion
  40 calories

Strawberry Compote

4 cups whole fresh or
  unsweetened fresh frozen
  strawberries
2 teaspoons unflavored
  gelatin
1 tablespoon fresh lemon
  juice
1 tablespoon fructose

1. Put the whole straw-
berries in a saucepan,
cover and cook over
very low heat for about
10 minutes.

2. Remove the lid and
bring to the boiling point.
Boil for 1 minute, remove
from the heat and set
aside.

3. Put the gelatin in the
lemon juice and let stand
for 5 minutes. Pour some
of the hot juice from the
strawberries into the
gelatin and stir until the
gelatin is completely
dissolved.

4. Add the dissolved
gelatin to the strawberries,
mix well and let cool to
room temperature.

5. Stir in the fructose and
refrigerate.

Variation Substitute any
fresh fruit for the strawberries.

Makes 3 cups
1/2 cup contains approximately:
  1 fruit portion
  40 calories

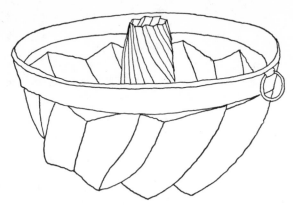

Ambrosia

2 envelopes (2 scant tablespoons) unflavored gelatin
1/4 cup cold water
1/4 cup water, boiling
3 cups sliced fresh or unsweetened fresh frozen
strawberries
One 8-ounce can crushed
pineapple in natural
juice, undrained
1 small banana, sliced
2 tablespoons fructose
1 teaspoon vanilla extract
1 teaspoon coconut extract
1/4 cup sour cream
1/4 cup plain low-fat yogurt

1. Soften the gelatin in the
cold water and allow to
stand for 5 minutes.

2. Add the boiling water
to the gelatin and stir until
the gelatin is completely
dissolved.

3. Put 2 cups of the strawberries, the dissolved gelatin, the pineapple and its
juice, banana, fructose,
vanilla and coconut ex-
tracts, sour cream and
yogurt in a blender con-
tainer and blend until
smooth.

4. Pour the mixture in a
bowl and add the remain-
ing 1 cup strawberries.
Mix well.

5. Spoon the mixture into
8 small soufflé dishes or
1 large dessert dish. Chill
until firm before serving.

Makes 8 servings
Each serving contains approximately:
1/4 fat portion
1 fruit portion
52 calories

Bananas North Pole

4 ripe bananas, peeled and
sliced
1 teaspoon freshly grated
orange peel
Fresh mint sprigs (optional)

1. Put the sliced bananas
in a plastic bag in the
freezer.

2. When the bananas are
completely frozen, put
them in a blender con-
tainer, a few at a time, and
blend just until smooth.

3. Spoon the frozen puréed
bananas into 8 sherbet
glasses and garnish with
orange peel and mint, if
available.

Makes 8 servings
Each serving contains approximately:
1 fruit portion
40 calories

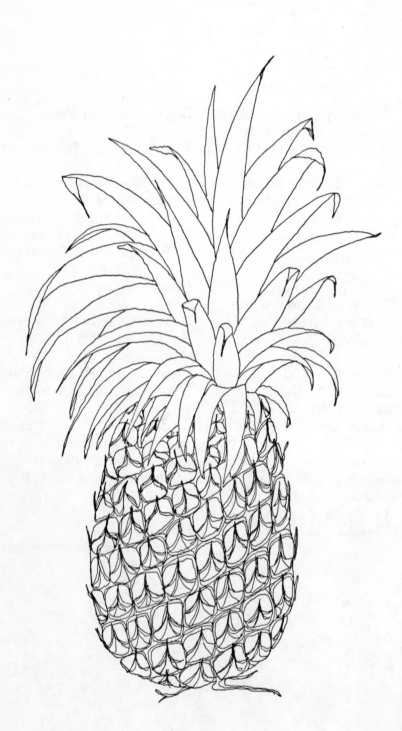

Pineapple Boats with Coconut Sauce

2 fresh pineapples
2 cups Coconut Sauce,
  following
Ground cinnamon

1. Cut the pineapples lengthwise into quarters, carefully cutting through the green leaves at the top to leave a section of leaves on each quarter.

2. Using a very small sharp paring knife, carefully cut the fruit from its shell. It is necessary to cut down both sides of the pineapple sections, beginning at the corners, to achieve this.

3. Cut off the hard core section at the top of each pineapple quarter and discard it.

4. Cut each pineapple quarter as it rests on its shell in half lengthwise, then cut it horizontally into bite-sized pieces.

5. To serve, top each pineapple boat with 1/4 cup Coconut Sauce and sprinkle lightly with cinnamon.

Makes 8 servings
Each serving contains approximately:
  1 fruit portion
  1/4 non-fat milk portion
  60 calories

Coconut Sauce

1 cup Jelled Milk, page 25
1 cup non-fat milk
1 teaspoon vanilla extract
1 teaspoon coconut extract

1. Put all of the ingredients in a blender container and blend until smooth.

2. Allow to stand a few minutes to thicken before serving.

Makes 2 cups
1/4 cup contains approximately:
    1/4 non-fat milk portion
    20 calories

Mango Whip

1 cup Jelled Milk, page 25
1 1/2 teaspoons fructose
1/2 teaspoon vanilla extract
1/2 cup non-fat milk, chilled
3 small ripe mangoes,
    peeled and diced

1. Put all of the ingredients in a blender container and blend on high speed for 2 minutes, or until very frothy.

2. Pour into 6 sherbet glasses and chill until set.

Note Instead of putting all of the diced mango in the blender container, some of it can be put in the bottom of each sherbet glass and the whipped mixture poured over it.

Fresh Peach Whip Variation Proceed as directed for Mango Whip, substituting 3 medium-sized peaches, peeled and diced, for the mangoes, 1/4 teaspoon almond extract for the vanilla extract, and reduce the fructose measure to 3/4 teaspoon.

Makes 6 servings
Each serving contains approximately:
    1/4 non-fat milk portion
    1 fruit portion
    60 calories

Blueberry Mousse

2 envelopes (2 scant tablespoons) unflavored gelatin
1/4 cup cold water
1/4 cup water, boiling
3 cups fresh or unsweetened fresh frozen blueberries
One 8-ounce can crushed pineapple in natural juice, undrained
1 teaspoon vanilla extract
1/2 cup plain low-fat yogurt
1/2 cup Whoopee Topping, page 75
Fresh mint sprigs (optional)

1. Soften the gelatin in the cold water and let stand for 5 minutes.

2. Add the boiling water to the gelatin and stir until the gelatin is completely dissolved.

3. Put 2 cups of the blueberries, the gelatin mixture, the crushed pineapple and its juice, vanilla extract, fructose and yogurt in a blender container and blend until smooth.

4. Pour the mixture in a bowl and add the remaining 1 cup blueberries. Mix well.

5. Spoon the mixture into 8 small soufflé dishes or 1 large dessert dish. Chill until firm before serving.

6. Top each serving with 1 tablespoon of Whoopee Topping. Garnish each with a mint sprig, if available.

Makes 12 servings
Each serving contains approximately:
    1 fruit portion
    40 calories

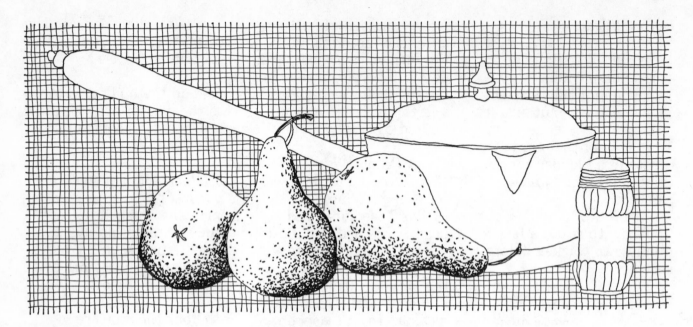

Poached Pears

8 firm ripe pears (Bartletts
  are best)
2 cups water
2 teaspoons vanilla extract
1 teaspoon rum extract
1/2 cup fructose
1/2 teaspoon ground
  cinnamon
1 cup Sauterne Sauce,
  following
Ground nutmeg

1. Peel the pears carefully,
leaving the stems on them.
With an apple corer, re-
move the cores from the
ends opposite the stems.

2. Put the water, vanilla,
rum extract, fructose and
cinnamon in a saucepan
and bring to a slow boil.

3. Place the pears in the
simmering water and cook,
turning frequently, about
10 minutes, or until easily
pierced with a fork but still
firm.

4. Remove the pears from
the heat and let cool to
room temperature in the
poaching liquid.

5. Cover and refrigerate
all day or overnight in the
liquid.

6. Place each pear on a
plate or in a shallow bowl
and spoon 2 tablespoons
Sauterne Sauce over the
top. Sprinkle each serving
with a touch of nutmeg.

Makes 8 servings
Each serving contains approximately:
  2 fruit portions
  1/2 fat portion
  103 calories

Sauterne Sauce

1/2 cup sour cream
1/2 cup plain low-fat yogurt
2 1/2 tablespoons sauterne

1. Combine all of the in-
gredients and mix well.

2. Cover and refrigerate
all day or overnight before
serving.

Makes 1 cup
2 tablespoons contain approximately:
  1/2 fat portion
  23 calories

82

Cold Orange Soufflé

2 envelopes (2 scant table-spoons) unflavored gelatin
1 cup cold water
2 egg yolks, at room temperature
Two 6-ounce cans frozen unsweetened orange juice concentrate, thawed
1 teaspoon vanilla extract
1/2 cup fructose
8 egg whites, at room temperature
1 cup skim evaporated milk, chilled
1 tablespoon freshly grated orange peel for garnish

1. Soften the gelatin in the cold water and let stand for 5 minutes.

2. Beat the egg yolks with an electric mixer or wire whisk until they are thick and foamy. Beat in the softened gelatin.

3. Pour the mixture into a saucepan and place over medium heat. Cook, stirring constantly, until thick enough to lightly coat a metal spoon. *Do not allow the mixture to come to a boil.*

4. Remove the pan from the heat and stir in the thawed orange juice concentrate, vanilla extract and fructose. Pour the mixture into a large mixing bowl and refrigerate until thickened to a syrupy consistency, about 20 minutes.

5. Beat the egg whites until they are stiff but not dry; set aside.

6. In another bowl, beat the chilled milk until it has quadrupled in volume.

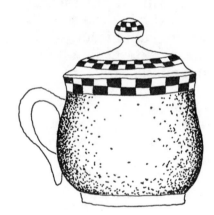

7. With a wire whisk, mix the whipped milk gently but thoroughly into the orange juice mixture.

8. Mix in the egg whites, gently folding them in until no streaks of white show.

9. Make a double-thickness waxed paper collar that will fit around the rim of a 7-inch (1 quart) soufflé dish. It should be wide enough to rise about 5 inches above the rim of the dish. Secure the collar to the dish with tape and then pour the soufflé mixture into the dish.

10. Refrigerate for at least 4 hours before removing the collar and serving the soufflé.

11. Lightly sprinkle the top with grated orange peel.

Makes 16 servings
Each serving contains approximately:
  1 1/4 fruit portions
  1/2 low-fat protein portion
  78 calories

Cheesecake

2 teaspoons corn oil
  margarine
4 graham cracker squares,
  crushed
2 cups (1 pint) low-fat
  small curd cottage cheese
1/4 cup liquid fructose
2 teaspoons vanilla extract
1 teaspoon freshly grated
  lemon peel
1 teaspoon fresh lemon
  juice

Topping
3/4 cup sour cream
2 tablespoons liquid
  fructose
1 1/2 teaspoons vanilla
  extract

1. Preheat the oven to
375°F.

2. Rub the 2 teaspoons of
margarine evenly over the
entire inner surface of a
9-inch pie plate.

3. Put the graham cracker
squares in a plastic bag
and roll them with a rolling
pin until they are fine
crumbs.

4. Sprinkle the crumbs
evenly over the greased pie
plate, pressing them down
with your fingertips to
make certain they stick to
the surface.

5. Put the cottage cheese,
fructose, vanilla extract
and lemon peel and juice in
a blender container and
blend until completely
smooth.

6. Pour the cottage cheese
mixture into the graham
cracker-lined pie plate and
spread it evenly.

7. Place the pie plate in the
center of the preheated oven
and bake for 15 minutes.

8. While the cheesecake is
baking, make the topping
by combining the sour
cream, liquid fructose and
vanilla extract in a bowl
and mixing well.

9. Remove the cheesecake
from the oven and spread
the topping evenly over
the surface. Return it
to the oven and bake for
10 more minutes.

10. Remove from the oven
and cool on a rack. Chill
thoroughly before serving.

Makes 16 servings
Each serving contains approximately:
  1/2 fat portion
  1/2 low-fat protein portion
  1/2 fruit portion
  71 calories

Eggnog Custard

4 eggs
4 cups non-fat milk
1/4 teaspoon salt
1/4 cup fructose
1 teaspoon ground
  coriander
2 teaspoons vanilla extract
1 teaspoon rum extract
Ground nutmeg

1. Preheat the oven to
250°F.

2. Put all of the ingre-
dients, except the nutmeg,
in a blender container and
blend well.

3. Pour the mixture into
a 6-cup baking dish and
sprinkle the top generously
with nutmeg.

4. Set the baking dish in
a shallow pan filled with
warm water and bake in
the preheated oven for
2 hours, or until the custard is set.

5. Cool to room tempera-
ture and then chill before
serving.

Makes 8 servings
Each serving contains approximately:
  1/2 medium-fat protein portion
  1/2 non-fat milk portion
  1/2 fruit portion
  97 calories

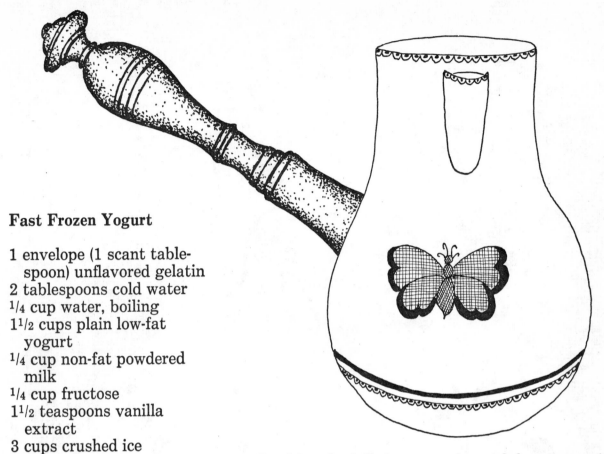

Fast Frozen Yogurt

1 envelope (1 scant tablespoon) unflavored gelatin
2 tablespoons cold water
1/4 cup water, boiling
1 1/2 cups plain low-fat
  yogurt
1/4 cup non-fat powdered
  milk
1/4 cup fructose
1 1/2 teaspoons vanilla
  extract
3 cups crushed ice

1. Soften the gelatin in the cold water and allow to stand for 5 minutes.

2. Add the boiling water to the gelatin and stir until the gelatin is completely dissolved.

3. Let the gelatin mixture cool to room temperature.

4. Combine the gelatin-water mixture with the yogurt and mix well. Refrigerate until firmly jelled.

5. Combine the jelled yogurt, milk powder, fructose, vanilla extract and crushed ice in a blender container and blend until smooth. Serve *immediately*.

Note   This is a sensational-tasting, soft frozen yogurt. Because the yogurt has never actually been frozen and processed, all of the valuable bacteria in it are still alive. You will also find that frozen yogurt is much less expensive when you make it yourself. You must serve it immediately, however. The taste diminishes rapidly and the good bacteria are killed off when it is frozen, and it becomes watery when stored in the refrigerator.

Makes 4 cups
1/2 cup contains approximately:
  1/4 low-fat milk portion
  1/2 fruit portion
  52 calories

85

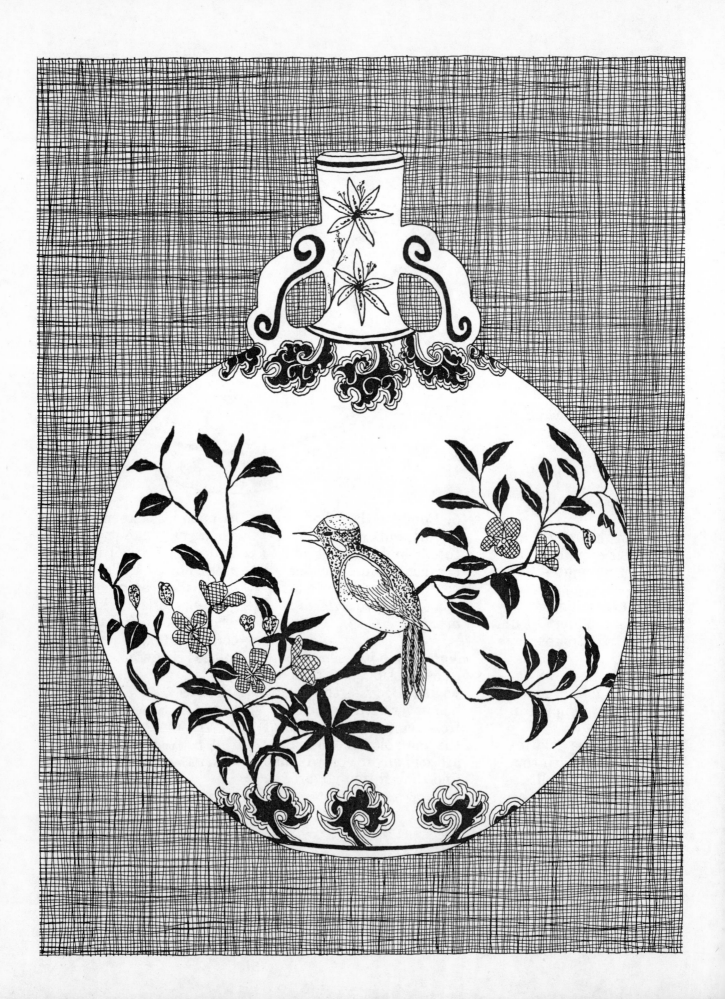

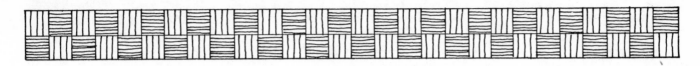

Beverages

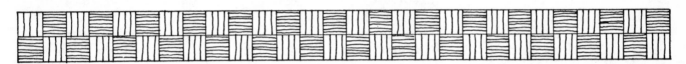

Appetite Appeaser

1/2 cup non-fat milk
2 teaspoons unprocessed
    wheat bran
1 1/2 teaspoons fructose

1. Put all of the ingredients in a blender container and blend until well mixed.

Note This Appetite Appeaser, taken one-half hour before mealtime, is helpful to many dieters in curbing appetite and making it easier not to overeat at mealtime. If using this during the first two-week program, omit the milk and 1/2 fruit portion from the following meal.

Makes 1 serving
One serving contains approximately:
  1/2 non-fat milk portion
  1/2 fruit portion
  60 calories

Sunrise Special

1/2 cup non-fat milk
1/2 cup fresh orange juice
1 tablespoon defatted
    wheat germ
1 tablespoon unprocessed
    wheat bran
1 tablespoon brewer's yeast
1/4 teaspoon vanilla extract
    (optional)
2 ice cubes, crushed
    (optional)

1. Put all of the ingredients in a blender container and blend until smooth and frothy.

Makes 1 serving
One serving contains approximately:
  1 fruit portion
  3/4 starch portion
  1/2 non-fat milk portion
  131 calories

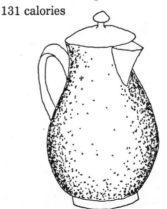

Banana Smoothie

1 small banana, sliced
1/2 cup non-fat milk
1/4 cup plain low-fat yogurt
1 teaspoon vanilla extract
Dash ground cinnamon
Ground cinnamon for
    garnish (optional)

1. Put all of the ingredients in a blender container and blend at high speed until smooth and frothy. Pour into a glass and garnish with cinnamon, if desired.

Note For a thicker smoothie, freeze the banana slices in a tightly closed plastic bag before preparing the drink.

Makes 1 serving
One serving contains approximately:
  2 fruit portions
  1/2 non-fat milk portion
  1/4 low-fat milk portion
  131 calories

White Eggnog

1 egg white
3/4 cup non-fat milk
1 teaspoon fructose
1/2 teaspoon vanilla extract
1/4 teaspoon rum extract
2 ice cubes, crushed
Ground nutmeg for garnish

1. Dip the whole egg, in the shell, in boiling water for 30 seconds.

2. Break the egg and put the egg white *only* in a blender container.

3. Add the milk, fructose, vanilla and rum extracts and ice cubes to the blender container and blend until smooth and frothy.

4. Pour into a large glass and sprinkle with nutmeg.

Makes 1 serving
One serving contains approximately:
   3/4 non-fat milk portion
   1/2 fruit portion
   1/4 medium-fat protein portion
   99 calories

Coffee Carob Cooler

1/2 cup non-fat milk
1 1/2 teaspoons carob powder
1/2 teaspoon instant coffee powder (regular or decaffeinated)
1/8 teaspoon ground cinnamon
1/4 teaspoon vanilla extract
1 1/2 teaspoons unprocessed wheat bran
1 1/2 teaspoons defatted wheat germ
1 1/2 teaspoons fructose
2 tablespoons low-fat small curd cottage cheese
2 ice cubes (optional)
Cinnamon stick for garnish (optional)

1. Put all of the ingredients in a blender container and blend until frothy.

Note   This is a deliciously different approach to breakfast. You get your coffee along with the rest of your breakfast in the same refreshing beverage. This is also a fast, nutritious approach to breakfast for people who are rushed in the morning.

Makes 1 serving
One serving contains approximately:
   1/2 non-fat milk portion
   1/2 starch portion
   1/2 fruit portion
   1/2 low-fat protein portion
   123 calories

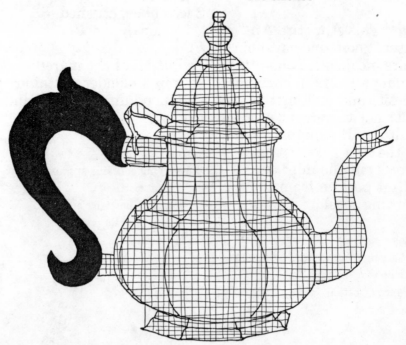

Peanut Butter Punch

1/2 cup non-fat milk
1 tablespoon unhomogen-
   ized peanut butter
1 1/2 teaspoons fructose
1/2 teaspoon unprocessed
   wheat bran
1/2 teaspoon vanilla extract
2 ice cubes
Ground cinnamon or nut-
   meg for garnish (optional)

1. Put all of the ingredients in a blender container
and blend until smooth and
creamy.

2. Pour into a chilled glass
and sprinkle a little cinnamon or nutmeg on the
top, if desired.

Note Peanut Butter
Punch is not only a deli-
cious and unusual bever-
age, but it also has a high
fiber content.

Makes 1 serving
One serving contains approximately:
   1/2 non-fat milk portion
   1/2 high-fat protein portion
   1/2 fruit portion
   108 calories

Paradise Punch

1/2 cup non-fat milk
1/2 cup unsweetened pine-
apple juice
2 tablespoons low-fat small
curd cottage cheese
1/2 teaspoon fructose
1/4 teaspoon vanilla extract
1/4 teaspoon coconut extract
2 ice cubes, crushed
(optional)

1. Put all of the ingredients in a blender container
and blend until smooth and
frothy.

2. Pour into a chilled glass
and serve.

Makes 1 serving
One serving contains approximately:
    1/2 non-fat milk portion
    1/2 low-fat protein portion
    1/2 fruit portion
    88 calories

Counterfeit Cocktail

Ice cubes
Perrier water or soda water
Fresh lime juice to taste
Angostura bitters

1. Fill a large wineglass
with ice cubes and Perrier
water and add lime and
2 dashes of Angostura bitters, or enough to make
the drink a beautiful pale
pink color.

Note This drink may be
prepared in a variety of
ways. It can be served in a
highball glass, a beer
mug—use your imagina-
tion. Most bars and cock-
tail lounges have all of the
ingredients, so you can
order it when you are dining out as well as prepare
it at home. It has a de-
cided advantage over most
non-alcoholic drinks in that
it is not sweet, the calories
are negligible and it is low
in sodium.

One 8-ounce serving contains ap-
proximately:
Free food
Calories negligible

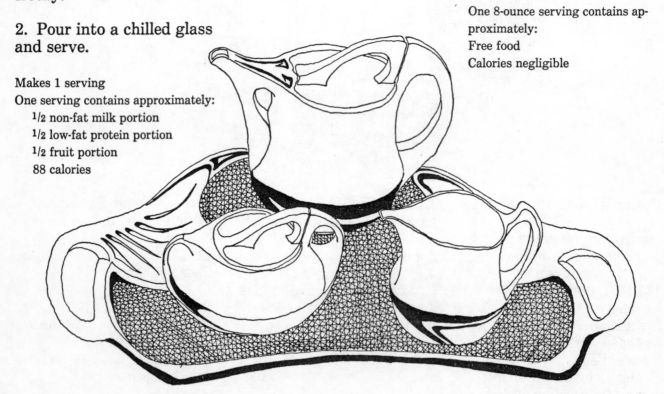

90

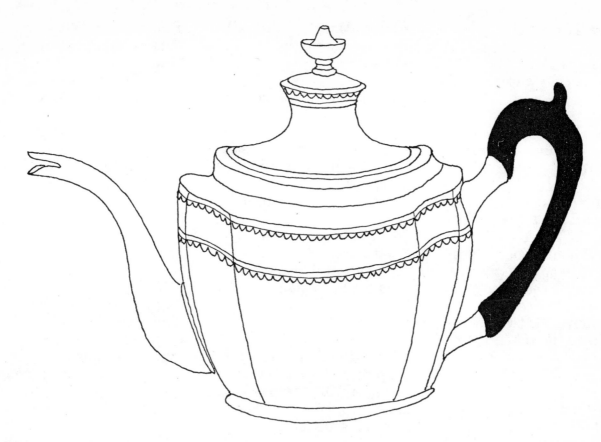

Calorie-Counter's Wine

Dry red, white or rosé wine
(amount desired)

1. Pour the wine into a non-aluminum saucepan and slowly bring to a boil.

2. When the wine starts to boil, ignite it with a match and allow it to burn until the flame goes out, thus burning off all of the alcohol. (Hold the lighted match with kitchen tongs that are at least 8 inches long, so you are not putting your hand close to the boiling wine when igniting it.) The volume of the wine will be reduced by the volume of the alcohol content of the wine.

3. Allow the wine to cool to room temperature, then store tightly covered in the refrigerator.

Note Wine with the alcohol removed is certainly not an epicurean delight, so using less expensive rather than valuable vintage wine is suggested. Removing the alcohol does, however, allow you to enjoy wine with your meals with reduced calories and no chance of a headache in the morning. Red wine is best served at room temperature and both white and rosé wines should be served chilled.

One 3-ounce serving contains approximately:
60 calories

Desert Tea

2 tea bags
2 quarts cold water

1. Put the tea bags in a 2-quart glass jar or bottle with a lid, fill with water and cover.

2. Put the jar in the sun until the tea is the desired strength. This usually takes 2 hours, sometimes more, depending upon the intensity of the sun.

3. Remove the tea bags and store the tea in the refrigerator.

Makes 8 servings
Each serving contains approximately:
Free food
Calories negligible

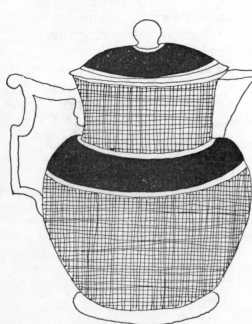

Bloody Mary (With Vodka)
Bloody Shame (Without Vodka)

1 teaspoon fresh lime juice
1/2 teaspoon Worcestershire sauce
1/4 teaspoon seasoned salt
Dash freshly ground black pepper
1 cup V-8 Juice or tomato juice
Dash Tabasco sauce (optional)
1 jigger (3 tablespoons) vodka (optional)
Ice cubes
Celery sticks

1. Mix the lime juice, Worcestershire sauce, seasoned salt and black pepper together until the salt is dissolved.

2. Add the V-8 or tomato juice and mix well. Add the Tabasco sauce and vodka, if desired.

3. Pour over ice and garnish with a celery stick for a stirrer.

Makes 2 servings
Each serving contains approximately:
1 vegetable portion
25 calories (without vodka)
125 calories (with vodka)

Ramos Fizz (With Gin)
Ramos Frappé (Without Gin)

3/4 teaspoon fructose
1 cup non-fat milk
1 teaspoon fresh lemon juice
1 teaspoon fresh lime juice
4 drops orange flower water
1 egg white
3 ice cubes, crushed
1 1/2 ounces gin (optional)
Ice cubes for serving
1/4 cup soda water

1. Put fructose, milk, lemon and lime juice, orange flower water, egg white, ice cubes and gin, if desired, in a blender container and blend until frothy.

2. Pour over ice in 2 tall glasses. Add 2 tablespoons of soda water to each glass and stir to mix.

Makes 2 servings
Each serving contains approximately:
1/2 non-fat milk portion
1/2 medium-fat protein portion
77 calories (without gin)
190 calories (with gin)

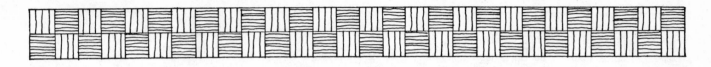

Exercise Program

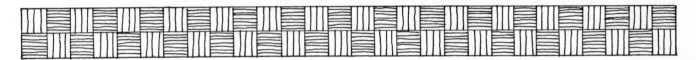

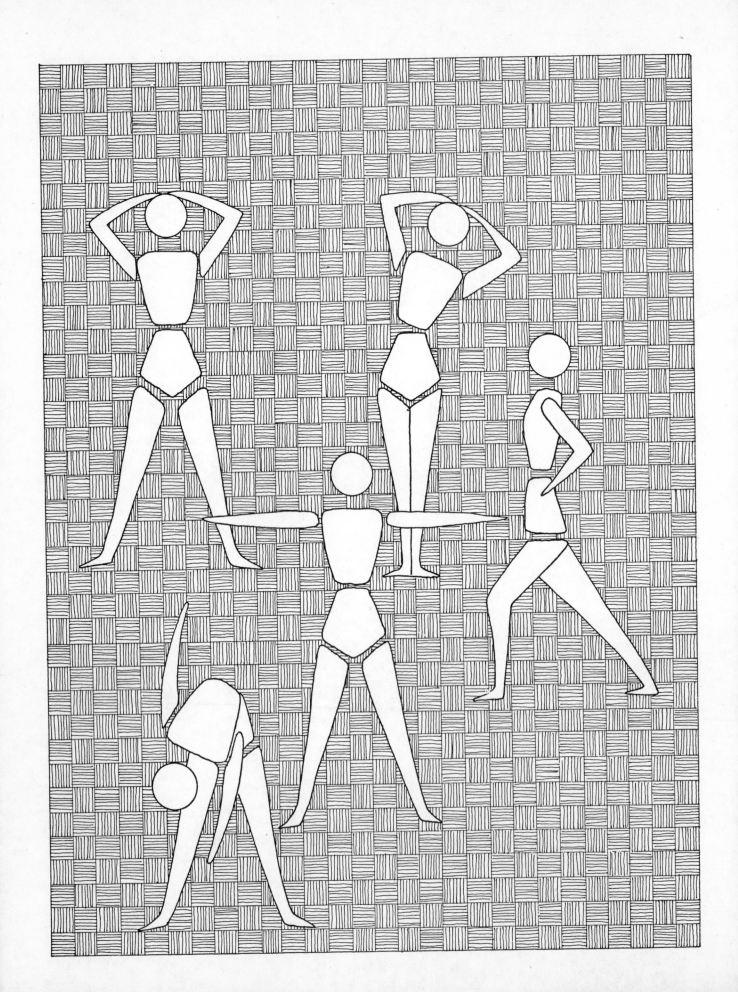

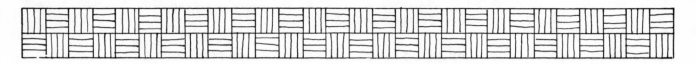

Fitness Is Fun

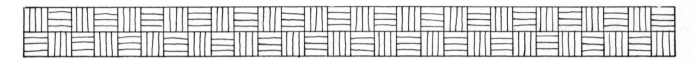

Exercise for Mind, Body and Spirit

Balancing your diet with exercise is the key to a successful fitness program—the key to a healthier, happier you. Why exercise?

Think of your body as an automobile. Of course you have to pour fuel into it, just as we give food to our bodies, to keep it running. And if you add a new coat of paint to the outside, your car will look great. But if you don't keep it tuned properly, you eventually will have to replace the entire automobile. We can't replace our bodies, but we can keep them in tune by proper eating, exercise and rest.

Exercise not only improves the way you look by burning off the calories you ingest, but it also improves the way you feel. By enhancing your circulation—pumping more oxygen into your brain—exercise also stimulates your intellect, your self-awareness and your productivity. Companies all over the world are offering fitness programs for their employees because studies show that 45 minutes of exercise a day can increase a person's productivity by four to five hours. You have more energy, tire less easily, are more mentally alert, more physically fit and therefore more capable of dealing with the tasks and problems that confront you.

Ultimately, a good fitness program will increase your self-respect, your self-confidence and the respect of others for you, because you stand taller, walk better, look radiant and think more clearly. Add it all together and it's fitness for a better body, mind and spirit.

Developing Your Personal Fitness Program

Fitness cannot be worked on one or two days a week. An effective exercise program must be a part of your daily regimen. In order to achieve this, you must first evaluate yourself and your life style, then motivate yourself, set goals and rewards, establish priorities, work out a schedule and choose those physical activities you enjoy most. You will soon learn that fitness can be fun—one of the greatest joys of your life.

Goals and Rewards

Set some specific goals for yourself, but be realistic and avoid crash programs. Don't hope to lose ten pounds in a week. You didn't put that weight on in a week, nor will you lose it in a week. You must change your life style and you will gradually see results. Your ultimate goal should be your overall appearance and well being—the shape you will be in a year from now.

You should also set immediate goals for daily or weekly improvements. During stretching exercises, for example, you will find a great sense of achievement in your daily progress if you work at it. When you bend over, maybe your fingers will only touch your knees the first day, but every day you will reach a few inches lower with ease. Charting your measurements, your heart rate and your weight periodically will heighten that sense of achievement as the changes become readily apparent.

In setting your goals, however, it is important to understand your body type. We are all born with a specific body type—whether mesomorph, ectomorph or endomorph—and there is nothing we can do to change certain things. Some people are just naturally thin, stocky, muscular, large busted or wide in the hip. You can't change the size of your bones or your metabolism. So be aware of these limitations and set your goals within them. You can, however, contour your body by working on specific areas you wish to improve.

The improved physical and mental state that fitness brings should be a sufficient reward in itself. But if you need other incentives, develop a reward system for yourself. Place your rewards on a graduated scale so you will always have something to look forward to and try to relate them to your goals. Buy a fancy new belt when you take two inches off your waist, splurge on a new dress when you lose that first ten pounds or promise yourself a vacation—perhaps even at a fitness, tennis or ski resort—if you've achieved your long-range goals in a year. One warning: Don't reward yourself with a double hot-fudge sundae or whatever your favorite food indulgence might be every time you lose another ten pounds. They might be the last you lose.

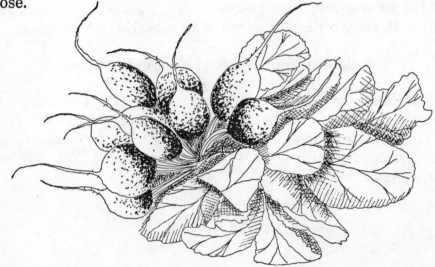

96

Priorities and Schedules

Make fitness high on the list of your daily priorities. Remember, when you say "I'll do it later," later never comes. Ideally you should set aside a specific time each day for fitness, stick to it and don't let yourself be interrupted. Learn to take the phone off the hook, if necessary, or put a Do Not Disturb sign on your door. There's also no such thing as "no time for fitness," because your new program will increase your productivity and enable you to accomplish much more in a shorter time than you did before.

Choosing the right time for your daily exercise routine depends completely on your schedule. Before breakfast is one of the best times, because you will feel more stimulated throughout the day. Or do your exercises on your lunch hour or before going to bed. In the evening, if you are tired and have to go out, a few simple exercises, some stretches and a shower will restore you so that you think you just took a long nap. In fact it's more beneficial for you than the nap.

If you have a family, get them to join you. Or if you feel silly doing a back rock stretch all by yourself in the office lunch room, organize your coworkers into a fitness class.

If circumstances on any given day interfere with your scheduled exercise period, don't worry. You can still do simple breathing, stretching and relaxation exercises while driving a car, sitting at a desk, watching television or when you get into bed at night. Learn to incorporate fitness and relaxation into every segment of your life.

Fitness Is Fun

Whatever your personal fitness program, keep it light and fun, something that you will look forward to doing every day. Accompany your stretching, breathing and relaxing exercises with the music you like best—whether disco or Debussy. The beat of the music will also help you establish a rhythm for your breathing and movements. And for your cardiovascular exercises, pick the activity you enjoy most—walking, jogging, swimming, tennis, aerobic dancing, or even skipping rope.

Safety First

It is wise to have a complete physical examination before starting any fitness program and to explain to your doctor what goals you hope to achieve and what type of exercises you will be doing. Your doctor can also help you determine a desirable weight level for your age, height and build. Take your measurements and learn to check your heart rate (see page 102) so you do not overexert. Wear comfortable clothing that does not restrict your movements—leotards and tights, shorts and a T-shirt, or even a bathing suit. And for walking, jogging and active sports, make sure you have supportive shoes. Finally, never push yourself too far. When you start to become tired or breathless, gradually slow down your pace and stop.

Caloric Intake and Energy Output

Exercise burns up calories. Thus in your fitness program you must always balance caloric intake against energy output. Stated very simply, if you wish to lose weight, you may do so by decreasing your caloric intake while maintaining a well-balanced diet and increasing your energy output through exercise. If you wish to maintain or gain weight, you should increase the number of calories in your diet to compensate for the energy expenditure.

There is no set formula regulating the number of calories a given exercise will burn up. This depends on your metabolism, your weight and how strenuously you pursue that exercise. The average 200-pound man, for example, might use up about 400 calories in an hour of calisthenics, whereas the average 125-pound woman would use only 250 calories. In a slow, hour-long walk, a 175-pound man would burn off about 240 calories, while his 150-pound companion would score less than 200. Even while you sleep you are burning calories, ranging from 40 for a 90-pound child to slightly over 100 for a 250-pound man.

14 Days to a New You

Our 14-day program is divided into two weeks. The first week begins with basic exercises, which increase in complexity and pace by the end of the week. The second week introduces a program designed for each part of the body—shoulders, waist, thighs, etc.—concentrating on a new part each day.

A total fitness program combines diet with four exercise components: stretching, breathing, relaxation and some form of more strenuous exercise, such as walking or swimming, to condition your cardiovascular system. But venturing into a new exercise program with cold muscles can cause you to cramp and feel total soreness. You should start slowly and warm up your body first, then increase your exercise experience each day. If possible, exercise in front of a mirror so that you can be sure that you are maintaining good posture.

Stretching

Stretching is the most important component in exercise, because as we become older our muscles become shorter and tauter and we lose our flexibility range if we don't keep them "stretched out." Without stretching we are more susceptible to knee, hip, shoulder and elbow injuries. While doing your stretching exercises, go slowly and gently at first. Do not strain your muscles beyond what you can do comfortably. If at first you can't touch your toes, don't worry. Reach as far as you can go—or bend your knees slightly. Later, as your muscles become more flexible, you will do these things easily.

Beside the stretching exercises in this book, there are many ways you may stretch throughout the day in the course of your normal activities. You can stretch in your automobile, aligning your spine against the car seat and readjusting your mirrors so that you have to sit tall to see out of them. You can stretch at your desk: Push your arms out straight against your desk and drop your head down between your arms. You can stretch when you reach down to a bottom drawer or up to a top shelf. You can stretch when you open a door: Instead of walking right up to the door handle, stop a little way off, flex your knees and reach out.

And there are countless ways you can stretch while watching television. In fact, most people could stay physically fit if they just incorporated stretching with watching TV. If you're sitting, raise your knees to your chest. If you're on the floor, rotate your legs from side to side, stretching overhead. Just crossing your arms and hugging yourself, trying to touch your shoulder blades, stretches your back.

If you are aware of yourself, stretching can be incorporated into everything you do.

Breathing

Proper breathing lets you perform the exercises you are doing with greater ease. Think of breathing as taking in fuel. You inhale, obtaining oxygen to keep alive; you exhale to push out all the "used air" in your lungs. But most of us neglect this part of exercising.

For a basic breathing exercise, place your hands over your rib cage or diaphragm. As you breathe in you should feel your diaphragm expanding like a balloon blowing up. When you think you have taken in all the air you can, breathe in a little more. This expands the diaphragm. When you exhale, you'll feel the ribs coming closer together and your abdominals contracting as if you're pressing all the air out of that balloon. When you think you have gotten all the air out, give it one more try with a little puff.

When doing your exercises, remember to inhale before beginning an exercise. Exhale when performing the most difficult or contracted stage of the exercise; inhale while returning to your starting position. Throughout the day, remember to walk tall and sit straight; your breathing will automatically improve. Constantly remind yourself to breathe deeply and regularly.

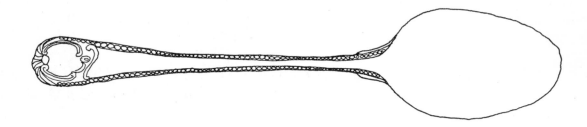

Walking

Walking is the most rewarding exercise that is good for everyone. In today's society we've all been told that jogging is excellent exercise. But in fact, jogging is on its way out because of the injuries and damages it can cause. Walking lets you exercise your whole body: your upper torso, your legs, your abdominals and your cardiovascular system—your heart.

Walking can be fun. Most people walk with their heads down and see nothing but cracks in the sidewalk and pebbles on the street. Most people walk with their heads forward, like their heads are trying to reach the destination before their bodies. They forget to roll their shoulders up to their ears and back and to elongate with their vortex, the very tip of the head. While you are walking, look to see the beautiful things around you. To give yourself a nice tall body and a good position to walk in, think of a plumb line dropping from the top of your head, down along your spine, through the back of your heels. Lift up your chest; contract your abdominal muscles and stretch them out at the same time. This very comfortable position also lets the pelvis tuck under where it belongs. Remember to keep your shoulders loose, rolling them up toward your ears and letting them drop down naturally and stay relaxed and low. Let your arms be loose and breathe in and out rhythmically as you're walking along.

A daily walk of eight to ten minutes to condition your cardiovascular system is part of your basic exercise program. You may substitute jogging, jumping rope or swimming if you have the facilities. But walking is good for everyone and can be done by everyone.

Before you go out on your walk, put on good supportive shoes. Take your pulse and chart your heart rate before starting (see page 103) so you can measure your cardiovascular progress. Then select a scenic route, if possible, and enjoy what you see. Start slowly at first, then gradually add briskness throughout the fitness program. But don't overextend your walk. And begin to slow down your pace a short distance from your home. You want a reduced heart rate for your relaxation period.

Relaxation

You won't get the total benefits from your fitness program if you don't incorporate relaxation exercises. These moments of silence will relax both your body and your mind. They will restore your system and prepare you for the day ahead.

Select a quiet place to do your relaxation exercises; turn on some quiet music. Then work to relax each part of the body totally. Slow movements. Rhythmic slow breathing. Breathing in new energy and exhaling used energy.

Throughout the day, whenever you feel tired or tense, take a few moments for relaxation. Lower your head, relax your shoulders, arms and hands, and breathe deeply. Or lie flat on the floor for a few moments with your knees bent and your palms stretched up and breathe deeply. You will be totally refreshed.

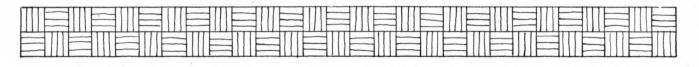

Basic Exercise Positions

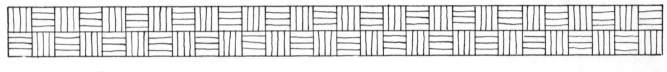

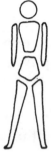

Basic Standing Position
Stand with a straight back, abdominals contracted, buttocks tucked under, soft knees and feet flat on the floor a hip width apart. Pull your shoulders up to your ears and roll them down.

Basic Sitting Position
Sit on the floor with a straight back, legs extended in front of body and hands beside hips for support.

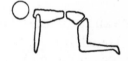

Basic Hands and Knees Position
Support yourself on your hands and knees, with a straight back, hands directly under shoulders, knees directly under hips and your weight evenly distributed on your hands and knees.

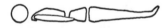

Basic Floor Position
Lie flat on your back on the floor, shoulders down, lower back in contact with the floor, arms at sides with palms down and legs extended.

Basic Stomach Position
Lie flat on your stomach on the floor, hips in contact with the floor, arms out at sides with palms up or down depending on the exercise, head to side and legs extended.

Basic Side Floor Position
Lie on your side on the floor, heels in line with buttocks, hip up toward ceiling, top arm in front for support and ear resting on extended lower arm.

Cardiovascular Conditioning/Aerobic Exercises

Cardiovascular or aerobic exercises strengthen the heart, enabling it to force the blood through the body slowly and steadily rather than in rapid, short pulsations that will wear it out. These exercises—swimming, bicycling, jumping rope, jogging, walking briskly—all require exertion. Your heart beats faster and you begin to breathe more deeply. The blood vessels expand, carrying oxygen and blood to your working muscles. When your body takes in more than the ordinary amount of oxygen you are burning calories more rapidly than normal. This continuous movement enables you to tone muscles and burn off fat at the same time. You should warm up slowly before any cardiovascular exercise or active sport, and you should always "walk it down"—bring down your level of exertion slowly rather than come to an abrupt halt.

The best way to measure your cardiovascular progress—and to be sure you don't overextend yourself—is by charting your heart rate or pulse. The lower your pulse, the more physically fit you are. Athletes, for example, have much lower pulses than average people.

Your maximum heart rate (beats per minute) decreases with age, as shown on the following Target Heart Rate Chart. It can be dangerous, however, to exceed 85 percent of your maximum rate and it is preferable to limit yourself to 75 percent of maximum for your age. This is called your target heart rate. Thus, by taking your pulse and charting your heart rate before, during and after strenuous exercise, you not only monitor the strengthening of your heart, but prevent yourself from straining it. As you become more fit, your resting heart rate should decrease and you should be able to exercise for longer periods before reaching your target rate.

Target Heart Rate

Age	Your maximum heart rate (beats/minute)	Your target heart rate (75% of the maximum in beats/minute)	Your target heart rate range (between 70–80% maximum in beats/minute)
20	200	150	140–170
25	195	146	137–166
30	190	142	133–162
35	180	139	130–157
40	180	135	126–153
45	175	131	123–149
50	170	127	119–145
55	165	124	116–140
60	160	120	112–136
65	155	116	109–132
70	150	112	105–128

Personal Heart Rate Chart

Date	1 Resting	2 Before Exercising	3 After Warmup	4 Cardio-vascular	5 End of Workout	6 After 3 Minutes

1. Resting heart rate is taken just before going to sleep, without any stimulants or depressants—coffee, tea, or alcohol, etc.—in your bloodstream. Feel your heart beat by holding your fingertips gently on the side of your neck or by holding them gently on the inside of your lower arm and count each beat as 1. Take your pulse for 10 seconds and multiply by 6.
2. Self-explanatory. Take your pulse for 10 seconds and multiply by 6.
3. Self-explanatory. Take your pulse for 10 seconds and multiply by 6.
4. Since the heart is a muscle, the cardiovascular time measurement refers to bringing the heart rate up to a target zone for the individual's heart to be exercised. This may be done by walking or participating in various sports. (See the section on cardiovascular conditioning on page 102.)
5. Self-explanatory. Take your pulse for 10 seconds and multiply by 6.
6. Three to five minutes after your workout, take your pulse for 10 seconds and multiply by 6 to see what your heart rate has returned to. This recovery rate should improve as you continue your routine workouts.

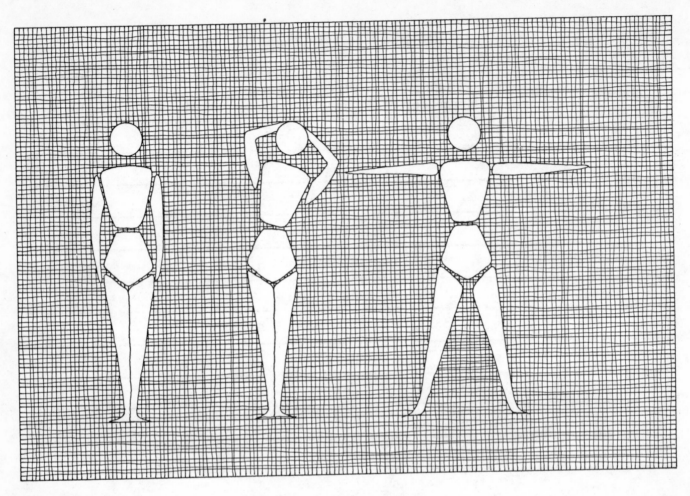

Charting Your Measurements

Jumping on the scales two or three times a day is a misinformed way to evaluate your total self. You may find your weight greater on one morning than on another simply because you finished your dinner late the preceding evening and it's still with you. Weighing daily can also be discouraging because weight loss should be gradual.

Instead, take your measurements before you start your fitness program and record them on your measurement chart. Then take them again every six weeks. Changes in specific measurements can be more indicative of physical fitness than overall weight loss or gain. In fact, you can improve your body and not lose any weight at all. Putting the weight in the right places is what counts. Muscle weighs more and takes up less space than fat. So you can reduce your dress or suit size drastically and maintain the same weight by converting that flabby fat into firm muscle through exercise.

When charting your measurements, always measure a relaxed muscle. For example, take the weight off your legs when measuring them: Sit down, rest one foot on a stool and measure your ankle, calf and thigh. Now repeat with the other leg.

104

Measurement Chart

Body Areas	First Week	Sixth Week	Twelfth Week	Eighteenth Week	Twenty-fourth Week
Waist					
Hips					
Lower Hips					
Thighs					
Bust					
Upper Left Arm					
Upper Right Arm					
Midriff					
Left Calf					
Left Ankle					
Right Calf					
Right Ankle					
Height					

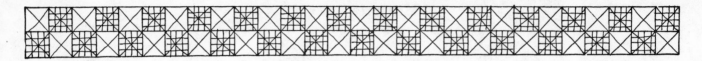

Glossary

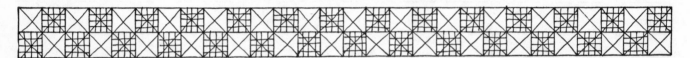

Abdominals
A span of muscles between the chest and pelvis. This is the largest span of muscles on the body that does not connect to bone. There are three major sets of abdominals: vertical, going vertically across the body; horizontal, going horizontally across the body; and diagonal, going diagonally across the body. Well-toned abdominals are important for good posture and for eliminating lower back pain.

Breathing
Important for achieving the most accomplished workout. Proper breathing permits us to exercise to the fullest potential. To breathe properly, think of your lungs as balloons. Blow up the "balloons" by inhaling as fully as you can, then breathe in a little more air so that you have the fullest inhalation possible. Then exhale, blowing out all of the air as though you are letting the balloons deflate. When you feel you have exhaled completely, force out a final little puff.

Buttocks
A very large, fleshy muscle, connected to the hips, on the backside of the body. One of the most difficult muscles to keep well toned.

Diaphragm
A body partition composed of muscle and connective tissue located just under the ribs. The diaphragm expands as we inhale and contracts as we exhale. To feel this movement, put one hand on either side of your rib cage just below the chest and breathe deeply.

Extension
The straightening out of a flexed limb to its fullest potential, thereby creating the most complete elongation of the muscle.

Flexion
The bending or flexing of a joint between the bones of a limb, thereby lessening the angle of the bones. For example, with arms outstretched, drawing your fingertips to your upper arms.

Pelvis
The area just below the abdominals and attaching to the hips. The pelvis, a structure of bone that houses vital organs, is a "free moving" area of the body. It is important to keep it in its proper position—tucked under and aligned with the legs and shoulders. Proper carriage of the pelvis is vital to good posture.

Pulse
When exercising, to gently "bounce" in the stated position to the count specified.

Roll down
Refers to lowering to the floor from a vertical sitting position to a completely supine position. To roll down properly, start the movement at the base of the tailbone with the pelvis tipped back and "roll down," one vertebra at a time, until your shoulders, and then finally your head, are in contact with the floor.

Roll up
Also round up, curl up. Refers to rising up to a vertical sitting position from a supine position. To "roll up" properly, tuck the chin and lift one vertebra at a time from the floor.

Shake out
Following an exercise, to relax that part of the body on which the exercise concentrated by freely shaking it, thereby relaxing the stretched muscles.

Thighs
The very large, powerful spans of muscle between the hips and knees. These are some of the most quickly toned muscles on the body and in turn must be kept long and lean by keeping them stretched. The thighs supply "drive" in specific exercises and play an important role in good posture.

Upper torso
The part of the body that is above the hips and reaches up into the shoulder area. During exercise, the upper torso can be isolated from the movement of the lower part of the body.

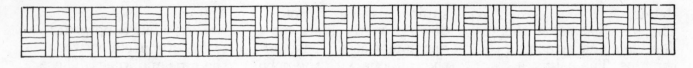

First Week Exercises

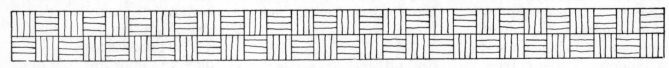

FIRST WEEK/DAY 1

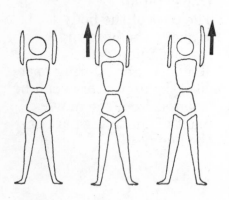

1. Overhead Stretch

a. Start in Basic Standing Position, with arms raised overhead. Be sure palms are in, pelvis is tucked under, abdominal muscles are contracted.
b. Reach right arm up, exhaling. Relax arm and inhale.

c. Reach left arm up, exhaling. Relax arm and inhale. Feel the total body stretch.
d. Repeat alternately 5 to 10 times on each side, exhaling as you reach up, inhaling as you relax your arms.
e. Shake out.

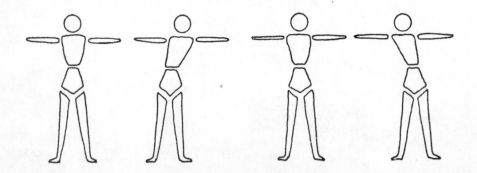

2. Side Stretch

a. Start in Basic Standing Position, with arms outstretched, palms down.

b. Without moving your hips, move your torso and reach to the right, exhaling as you go.
c. Inhaling, return to the starting position.
d. Exhaling, reach left. Then inhaling, return to the starting position.

e. Repeat alternately 7 times on each side, exhaling as you reach, inhaling as you relax.
f. Shake out.

3. Leg Stretch

a. Start in Basic Standing Position, with hands on hips and a tall spine. Inhale.
b. Move you right leg forward, and exhaling, slowly bend your right knee, keeping feet straight forward, heels down. Slowly move your pelvis forward until your knee obscures your foot.
c. Hold this stretch for 5 to 10 seconds, breathing evenly.
d. Repeat 4 times on each side.
e. Shake out.

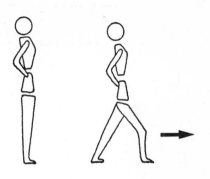

---

4. Walk or other cardiovascular exercise 5 to 10 minutes. Remember to chart your heart rate.

---

5. Relaxation: Sit and Reach Stretch

a. Start in Basic Sitting Position, with legs extended, arms on your knees. Inhale.
b. Exhaling slowly, slide your hands down your legs as far as you can reach comfortably. Tuck in your chin, round your back and contract your abdominal muscles. Reach for your ankles and hold 5 seconds, breathing evenly.
c. Inhaling, slowly return to the starting position.
d. Repeat 8 to 10 times.

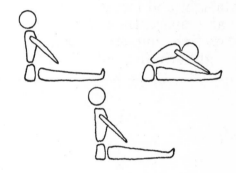

---

6. Basic Relaxation Exercise

a. Start in Basic Sitting Position, with knees bent.
b. Exhaling, slowly roll down to the floor, one vertebra at a time, until you are lying on the floor.
c. Let your spine come in contact with the floor, feet in line with your hips, arms outstretched, eyes closed. Rest until you feel relaxed.
d. Practice relaxation explained on page 100.

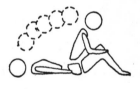

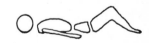

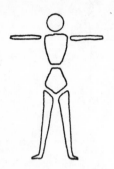 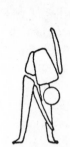 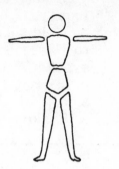 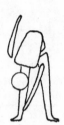

1. Cross Over Toe Touch
a. Start in Basic Standing Position, with arms outstretched at shoulder height and feet comfortably apart. Inhale.
b. Exhaling, cross your right arm in front of your body and touch the toes of your left foot.
c. Inhaling, return to the starting position.
d. Exhaling, cross your left arm in front of your body and touch the toes of your right foot.
e. Inhaling, return to the starting position.
f. Repeat alternately 5 times on each side. If you have difficulty reaching your toes, relax your knees slightly.
g. Shake out.

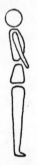 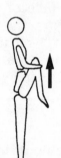 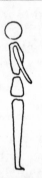 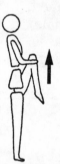

2. Knee to Chest Stretch

a. Start in Basic Standing Position. Inhale.
b. Exhaling, slowly raise your right knee to your chest and hold it with both hands. Pull to chest.
c. Inhale. Slowly return to the starting position. Inhale again.
d. Exhaling, repeat on the left side. Feel your total body stretch and keep a tall spine.
e. Repeat alternately 5 to 10 times on each side.
f. Shake out.

3. Swing Through

a. Start in Basic Standing Position, with feet outside hip line.
b. Inhaling, reach up with your right hand.
c. Keeping your right hand up, reach up with your left hand and touch your hands together.

d. Exhaling, slowly swing your hands between your legs, keeping your knees flexed (bent), back rounded, chin tucked in. Return to the starting position.
e. Repeat 10 times. Remember to exhale when you swing forward.
f. Shake out.

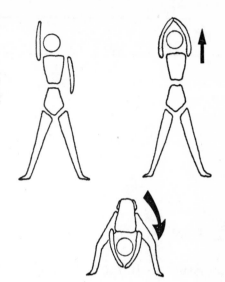

---

4. Walk or other cardiovascular exercise 5 to 10 minutes.

---

5. Relaxation: Back Rock Stretch

a. Start in Basic Sitting Position, with legs extended. Inhale.

b. Bend your knees up, feet flat. Take hold of the backs of your thighs, chin tucked in, back rounded.

c. Exhaling, slowly rock back and forth.
d. Repeat 8 to 10 times or more. Feel the massage along your spine.

---

6. Basic Relaxation Exercise

a. Start in Basic Sitting Position, with knees bent.
b. Exhaling, slowly roll down to the floor, one vertebra at a time, until you are lying on the floor.

c. Let your spine come in contact with the floor, feet in line with your hips, arms outstretched, eyes closed. Rest until you feel relaxed.
d. Practice relaxation explained on page 100.

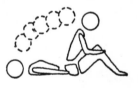

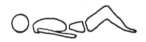

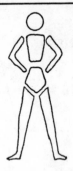 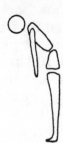

1. Back Stretch

a. Start in Basic Standing Position, with hands on hips. Inhale.

b. Exhaling, bend forward toward your toes, with your chin tucked in.

c. Bend your knees, round your back and, inhaling slowly, return to the starting position.
d. Repeat 5 to 10 times.
e. Shake out.

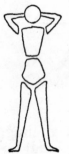 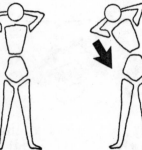 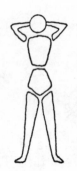 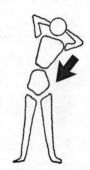

2. Side Waist Bend

a. Start in Basic Standing Position, with arms behind ears. Inhale.

b. Exhaling slowly, bend at your waist toward the right side (do not lean forward or backward).
c. Tighten your abdominal muscles and buttocks and, inhaling, return to center.

d. Repeat the above move to the left side.
e. Repeat alternately 10 to 15 times on each side.
f. Shake out.

3. Hip Twist

a. Start in Basic Standing Position, with arms outstretched. Inhale.
b. Shift weight to your left leg, bend your right knee and, exhaling, rotate the right knee across the left support leg, twisting your right hip forward and keeping your right toe on the floor.

c. Inhaling, turn your right knee out, rotating the whole leg and hip out.
d. Continue rotating 8 to 10 times, exhaling as you cross over, inhaling as you rotate out. Repeat with left knee. Keep tall and keep your abdominal muscles and buttocks contracted.

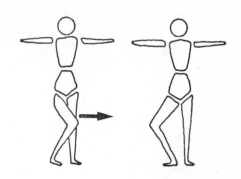

---

4. Walk or other cardiovascular exercise 5 to 10 minutes, increasing your pace over the previous day's. Remember to check your heart rate.

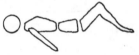 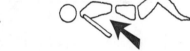 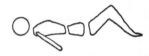

5. Relaxation: Pelvis Rock

a. Start in Basic Floor Position, with knees bent and arms outstretched.
b. Exhaling, contract your abdominal muscles, tipping your pelvis back so your total spine is in contact with the floor.
c. Inhaling, let your pelvis rock forward, leaving your buttocks on the floor. You will feel a little tunnel under your lower back.
d. Repeat 10 to 15 times, exhaling as you rock back, inhaling as you rock forward. Don't be in a hurry to finish this relaxation exercise.

---

6. Basic Relaxation Exercise

a. Start in Basic Sitting Position, with knees bent.
b. Exhaling, slowly roll down to the floor, one vertebra at a time, until you are lying on the floor.
c. Let your spine come in contact with the floor, feet in line with your hips, arms outstretched, eyes closed. Rest until you feel relaxed.
d. Practice relaxation explained on page 100.

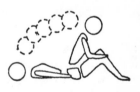

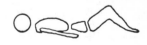

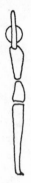
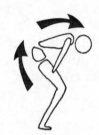
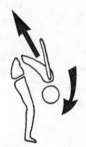

1. The Swing

a. Start in Basic Standing Position, with arms raised overhead and palms in. Reach tall overhead and inhale.

b. Swing arms down slowly behind your thighs, exhaling. Tuck in your chin and flex your knees.
c. Straighten your knees and reach your arms behind. Swing forward.

d. Return to the starting position.
e. Repeat 8 to 10 times. Feel the free swinging motion.
f. Shake out.

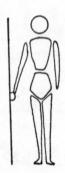
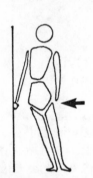
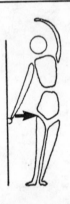

2. Waist Stretch

a. Start in Basic Standing Position, holding onto a bar or door knob with your right hand. Inhale.
b. Exhaling, let your right hip lean into the wall or door, dropping your left

arm down toward your feet.
c. Inhaling, slowly raise your left arm up and over your head, palm up, letting your hip stretch away from the wall or door, feeling the total stretch.

d. Exhaling, lower your arm and again stretch your hip toward the wall.
e. Repeat 10 times on each side, exhaling as you stretch toward the wall, inhaling as you stretch away.
f. Shake out.

3. Abdominals

a. Start in Basic Floor Position, with knees bent, feet flat, arms along your sides. Inhale.

b. Exhaling, contract your abdominal muscles. Lift your head and reach for your knees. Hold 4 counts, breathing evenly.

c. Inhaling, return to the starting position, keeping your lower back in contact with the floor.

d. Repeat 10 times, exhaling as you rise, inhaling as you recline.

e. Shake out.

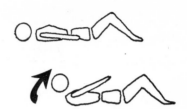

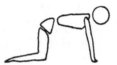 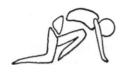

4. Donkey Kick

a. Start in Basic Hands and Knees Position, with back straight and abdominal muscles contracted. Inhale.

b. Exhaling, round your back, draw one knee up to your chest and tuck in your chin. Feel the energy in the knee coming in.

c. Inhaling, swing your leg back as far as you can and raise your head.

d. Exhaling, swing your knee forward to your chest again, tucking in your chin.

e. Repeat 6 to 8 times on each side.

f. Shake out.

5. Scissors Kicks

a. Start in Basic Side Floor Position, with toes pointed.

b. Open and close both legs, crossing your top leg over your bottom leg in a scissors motion parallel with the floor. Keep your hip toward the ceiling, abdominal muscles contracted. Reach away with pointed toes to get a long stretch.

c. Repeat 20 times on each side.

d. Shake out.

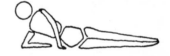

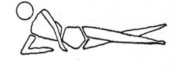

6. Walk or other cardiovascular exercise 5 to 10 minutes, increasing the briskness of the activity. Remember to check your heart rate.

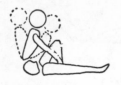

7. Relaxation: Hip Stretch

a. Start in Basic Sitting Position.
b. Bend your left leg, putting your left foot in your right hand or the bend of your right arm. Wrap your left arm around your thigh and cradle your leg.
c. Breathing rhythmically, rock gently back and forth.
d. Exhale and feel the tension disappear.

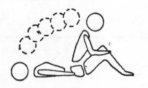
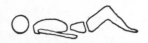

8. Basic Relaxation Exercise

a. Start in Basic Sitting Position, with knees bent.
b. Exhaling, slowly roll down to the floor, one vertebra at a time, until you are lying on the floor.
c. Let your spine come in contact with the floor, feet in line with your hips, arms outstretched, eyes closed. Rest until you feel relaxed.
d. Practice relaxation explained on page 100.

FIRST WEEK/DAY 5

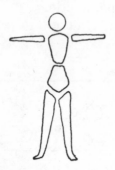
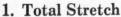
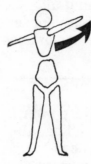
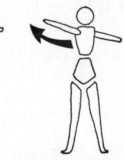

1. Total Stretch

a. Start in Basic Standing Position, with arms outstretched. Inhale.
b. Exhaling, look over your right shoulder, leading around with your right arm and with the left following. Feel the total stretch.
c. Inhale. Start the return action by looking over your left shoulder, exhaling and rotating to the left side.

Your total body will start to warm up, and by leading with your eyes, you also work on your neck, eyes and chin areas.
d. Repeat 20 times, working up to 35.
e. Shake out.

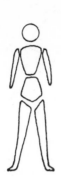 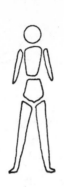 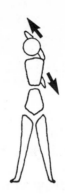

2. Side Bend

a. Start in Basic Standing Position. Inhale.
b. Exhaling, bring your right arm overhead and your left arm behind your back. Look over your left

shoulder, stretching both arms in opposite directions and keeping your body in line, not bending forward or backward.
c. Inhaling, return to the Basic Standing Position.

d. Exhaling, repeat on the opposite side, bringing your left arm overhead and completing the stretch as done on your right side.
e. Repeat alternately 10 to 15 times on each side.
f. Shake out.

 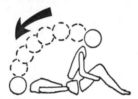 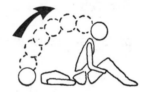 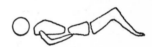

3. Situps

a. Start in Basic Sitting Position, with knees bent and back rounded. Inhale.
b. Exhaling, slowly roll down, one vertebra at a time, chin tucked in and

back rounded, until you are lying on the floor. Inhale.
c. Exhaling, tuck your chin in and return to the starting position, one vertebra at a time. (If you have difficulty coming up to the starting position,

bend your elbows and put your hands, palms down, by the small of your back, then push yourself up one vertebra at a time.)
d. Repeat 10 times, building up to 20 times.
e. Shake out.

---

4. Side Leg Lift

a. Start in Basic Side Floor Position. Inhale.
b. Exhaling, lift up your top leg about 12 inches, leading with your heel and with your foot flexed.

c. Inhaling, lower your leg very slowly.
d. Repeat 10 to 15 times on each side.
e. Shake out.

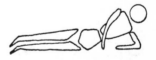
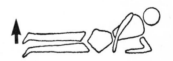

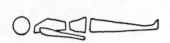 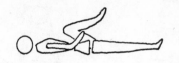 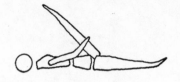

5. Leg Stretch

a. Start in Basic Floor Position. Inhale.
b. Exhaling, draw your left knee to your chest,

holding onto the back of your thigh. Pulse 4 times in this position, breathing evenly.
c. Exhaling, straighten your leg, holding onto the

back of your thigh. Pulse 4 times, breathing evenly.
d. Return to the bent knee position and repeat 6 to 8 times with each leg.
e. Shake out.

---

6. Walk or other cardiovascular exercise 5 to 10 minutes. Remember to breathe rhythmically.

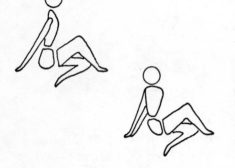

7. Relaxation: Cross Leg Stretch

a. Sit with your left leg bent in. Cross your right leg over your left leg. Place your left hand on your right knee and your right hand on the floor for support. Inhale.

b. Exhaling, rotate your upper body to your right, looking over your right shoulder.
c. Hold this position 10 seconds, breathing evenly and exhaling.
d. Return to the starting position and repeat 4 to 6 times on each side.
e. Shake out.

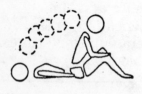

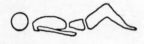

8. Basic Relaxation Exercise

a. Start in Basic Sitting Position, with knees bent.
b. Exhaling, slowly roll down to the floor, one vertebra at a time, until you are lying on the floor.

c. Let your spine come in contact with the floor, feet in line with your hips, arms outstretched, eyes closed. Rest until you feel relaxed.
d. Practice relaxation explained on page 100.

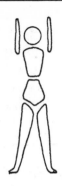   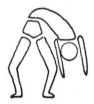

1. Stretch Swing (The figure shows a rounded back and flexed knee position. This exercise may be done with your legs straight as you continue to progress.)

a. Start in Basic Standing Position, with arms raised overhead. Extend your total body, keeping your abdominals contracted and your buttocks tucked under.
b. Exhaling, bend down to your right side. Contract your abdominal muscles and pulse several times, breathing rhythmically.
c. Without standing up, move to your left. Pulse several times, breathing rhythmically and keeping your abdominal muscles tight.
d. With your knees flexed, round your back and slowly return to the starting position.
e. Repeat 8 to 10 times, or until your muscles feel limber.
f. Shake out.

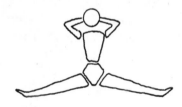 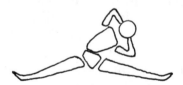 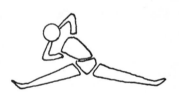

2. Sitting Waist Stretch

a. Start in Basic Sitting Position, with legs in a V position, a tall spine and your hands clasped behind your ears.
b. Exhaling, bend your left elbow to the floor outside your left knee as far down as your muscles are able to go without straining. Keep your back straight and your chin tucked in.
c. Hold this position for 10 to 15 seconds, breathing evenly.
d. Inhaling, return to the starting position.
e. Repeat the above move, going to your right side.
f. Repeat alternately 8 to 10 times on each side.
g. Shake out.

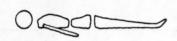 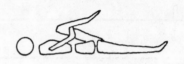

3. Abdominals

a. Start in Basic Floor Position, with legs extended and lower back pressed to the floor. Inhale.

b. Exhaling, contract your abdominal muscles and draw your right knee to your chest. Inhale.
c. Exhaling, simultaneously extend your right leg and draw in your left knee.
d. Do 20 alternate moves. Be sure to keep your lower back pressed to the floor.
e. Shake out.

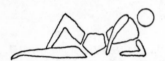

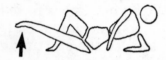

4. Inner Thigh Lift

a. Start in Basic Side Floor Position, with top leg bent, bottom leg straight with foot flexed, and hips as far forward as possible.
b. Keeping the foot flexed, slowly lift and lower the straight leg, feeling the energy in the heel. Keep your abdominal muscles contracted.
c. Repeat 10 times on each side.
d. Shake out.

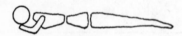

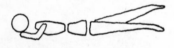

5. Back of Leg and Buttocks

a. Start in Basic Stomach Position, with hips flat on the floor and arms crossed and supporting your chin. Inhale.
b. Keeping your hips on the floor, tighten your buttocks and the backs of your legs, toes pointed.
c. Exhaling, slowly lift up one leg, then, inhaling, slowly lower it.
d. Repeat 10 times on each side, remembering to keep your hips down and abdominal muscles contracted.
e. Shake out.

6. **Walk** or other cardiovascular exercise 5 to 10 minutes.

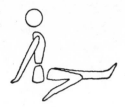 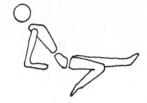 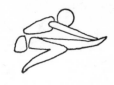

7. Relaxation: Sitting Thigh Stretch

a. Start in Basic Sitting Position, with hands behind your back.
b. Bend your right leg

back, supporting yourself on your hands. Inhale.
c. Exhaling, lower to your forearms, tipping your pelvis back. Hold for 4 counts, breathing evenly.
d. Exhaling, raise up, stretch forward and reach

straight out for your toes. Hold for 4 counts, breathing evenly.
e. Repeat this back stretch and forward reach 4 times on each side, moving slowly and breathing evenly.

8. Basic Relaxation Exercise

a. Start in Basic Sitting Position, with knees bent.
b. Exhaling, slowly roll down to the floor, one vertebra at a time, until you are lying on the floor.

c. Let your spine come in contact with the floor, feet in line with your hips, arms outstretched, eyes closed. Rest until you feel relaxed.
d. Practice relaxation explained on page 100.

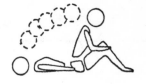

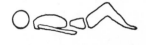

FIRST WEEK/DAY 7

1. Elbow to Knee Stretch

a. Start in Basic Standing Position, with elbows bent and hands at shoulder height. Inhale.
b. Exhaling, raise your left knee and lower your right elbow until they touch.

c. Inhaling, return to the starting position and transfer your weight to your left leg.
d. Exhaling, raise your right knee and lower your left elbow until they touch.
e. Repeat alternately 8 times on each side.
f. Shake out.

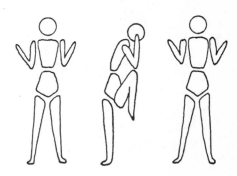

121

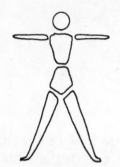 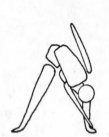 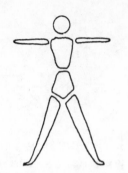 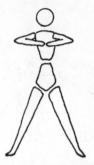 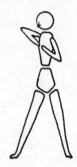

2. Bent Knee Toe Touches and Waist Turn

a. Start in Basic Standing Position, with feet comfortably apart outside hip line and arms outstretched. Inhale.

b. Exhaling, bend your left knee and cross over with your right hand. Pulse 1 or 2 times.
c. Inhaling, slowly return to the starting position.
d. Bend your elbows until your fingertips touch, look over your right shoulder

and, exhaling, turn back, leading with your right elbow. Pulse 1 or 2 times. Keep your hips locked forward, working your waistline.
e. Repeat 8 to 10 times on each side.
f. Shake out.

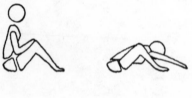
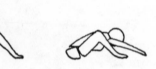
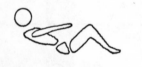

3. Abdominal Stretch and Tuck

a. Start in a sitting position, with feet flat on the floor, legs apart and hands on knees. Inhale.
b. Exhaling, stretch your hands and head through your legs, with chin tucked in. Pulse 4 times.
c. Inhaling, slowly come

back and then exhale. Contract your abdominal muscles and tuck your pelvis under (flattening the abdominal area). Keep your arms outstretched, palms up. Pulse 4 times.
d. Repeat the forward stretch and back tuck 10 to 20 times. Remember to breathe.
e. Shake out.

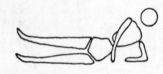
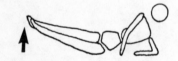

4. Inner Thigh

a. Start in Basic Side Floor Position, with top leg raised. Inhale and point toes.
b. Exhaling, lift your bot-

tom leg to meet your top leg.
c. Inhaling, lower your bottom leg, leaving your top leg up.
d. Repeat 6 to 8 times on each side.

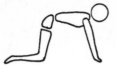 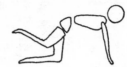 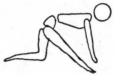

5. Hydrant

a. Start in Basic Hands and Knees Position, with abdominal muscles contracted. Inhale.
b. Exhaling, lift your right leg up and out to the side.

Energy is in your outer knee for lift. Look over your right shoulder and see your knee and ankle. Breathe evenly.
c. Exhaling, contract your abdominal muscles and ex-

tend your right leg straight out to the side.
d. Inhaling, bend your knee and return to the starting position.
e. Repeat 4 times on each side, building up to 8 to 10 times.

---

6. Walk or other cardiovascular exercise 5 to 10 minutes, trying to go the same distance in less time.

---

7. Relaxation: Back Stretch

a. Start in a cross-legged sitting position, with hands on knees. Inhale.
b. Exhaling, gently bend forward. Tuck in your chin and feel the long comfor-

table stretch. Place your hands on the floor in front of your head.
c. Hold 8 to 10 seconds, breathing evenly.
d. Inhaling, slowly roll up to the starting position.
e. Repeat 4 to 6 times.

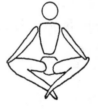

---

8. Basic Relaxation Exercise

a. Start in Basic Sitting Position, with knees bent.
b. Exhaling, slowly roll down to the floor, one vertebra at a time, until you are lying on the floor.

c. Let your spine come in contact with the floor, feet in line with your hips, arms outstretched, eyes closed. Rest until you feel relaxed.
d. Practice relaxation explained on page 100.

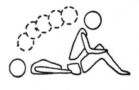

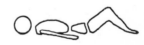

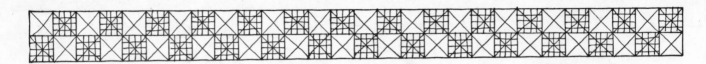

Second Week Exercises: Spot Control

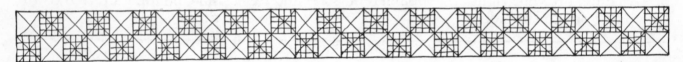

After the first week of the *Fitness First* program, your body should be in better shape overall—your muscles more flexible, your endurance better, your tensions eased, your weight a little more to your liking. The exercises for the second week are devoted to working on specific parts of your body, starting with the neck and shoulders on the first day and working down to the legs on the seventh day, according to the following schedule:

Day 1: Neck and Shoulders
Day 2: Arms, Upper Back and Chest
Day 3: Waist
Day 4: Abdominals and Lower Back

Day 5: Hips
Day 6: Inner and Outer Thighs
Day 7: Legs and Feet

Before doing any of the spot control exercises, *it is extremely important that you warm up* with three to five minutes of stretching exercises from the first week of the *Fitness First* program. In the future use these spot control exercises to reduce and contour various parts of your body that need working on. If you're too fat—or too thin—in the thighs, for example, concentrate on thigh exercises daily. Excess fat will gradually turn into lean muscle. Or, if you have skinny thighs, the developing muscles will start to fill them out. It works both ways.

Massage is also helpful for spot control. You can break down fat deposits in a particular area by kneading it with your hands, as you would bread, when you bathe or shower. Or rub your body with your hands or a loofa sponge. Massaging your body regularly will also help to relax tired or sore muscles.

Warm up with 3 to 5 minutes of stretching from the first week's program.

1. Neck I

a. Start in a cross-legged sitting position, with hands on knees. Inhale.
b. Exhaling, slowly drop your right ear to your right shoulder. Inhale on the return. Feel the stretch in the side of your neck.
c. Repeat the move, dropping your left ear to your left shoulder.
d. Repeat alternately 5 times on each side, working up to 10.

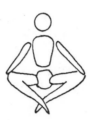 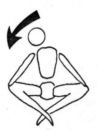

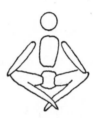 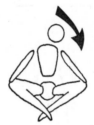

2. Neck II

a. Start in Basic Sitting Position, with ankles crossed and abdominal muscles contracted.
b. Exhaling, slowly let your head drop back, feeling the stretch from the chin down. Open your mouth and move your lower jaw up and down 6 to 8 times, raising your chin slightly each time. Remember to keep a tall back and your abdominal muscles tight.
c. Exhaling, slowly bring your head forward and down, chin tucked in, keeping your back tall and feeling the stretch in the back of your neck.
d. Repeat 8 times.

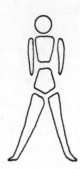 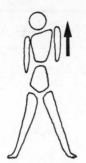 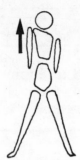

3. Shoulders I

a. This exercise may be done in Basic Standing or Sitting Position. Be comfortable. Inhale.

b. Lift your left shoulder toward your left ear, exhaling. Keep your abdominal muscles contracted and your spine tall.

c. Inhaling, lower your shoulder to the starting position.
d. Repeat 10 times on each side. You can vary the exercise by alternating sides.
e. Shake out.

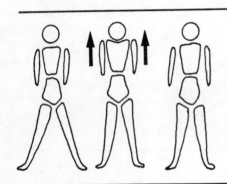

4. Shoulders II

a. This exercise may be done in Basic Standing or Sitting Position.
b. Lift both shoulders toward your ears, exhaling.

c. Lower your shoulders, to the starting position, inhaling. Keep your abdominal muscles contracted and your spine tall and move smoothly.
d. Repeat 10 times.
e. Shake out.

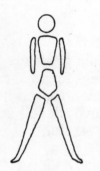 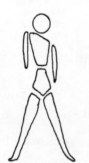 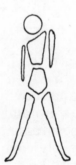

5. Shoulders III

a. This exercise may be done in Basic Standing or Sitting Position.
b. Move your shoulders, one at a time, forward. The move should form a complete circle. Breathe rhythmically and think of forming the letter "O."
c. Complete 10 circles forward with each shoulder, then reverse and roll backward 10 times.
d. Shake out.

6. Walk or other cardio-vascular exercise 8 to 10 minutes. Remember to chart your heart rate.

7. Basic Relaxation Exercise

a. Start in Basic Sitting Position, with knees bent.
b. Exhaling, slowly roll down to the floor, one vertebra at a time, until you are lying on the floor.

c. Let your spine come in contact with the floor, feet in line with your hips, arms outstretched, eyes closed. Rest until you feel relaxed.
d. Practice relaxation explained on page 100.

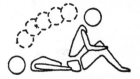
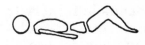

SECOND WEEK/DAY 2: ARMS, LOWER BACK AND CHEST

Warm up with 3 to 5 minutes of stretching from the first week's program.

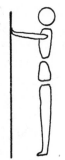
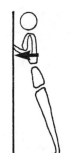
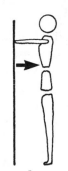

1. Upper Back/Chest

a. Start in Basic Standing Position, with your hands on the wall at chest level, fingertips pointing inward.

b. Slowly bend your elbows and lower yourself to the wall. Keep your body straight from your shoulders to your heels.

c. Slowly push away from the wall.
d. Repeat 20 times.
e. Shake out.

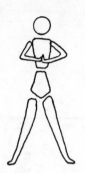 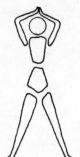 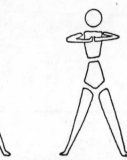 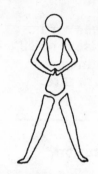

2. Chest Press

a. Start in Basic Standing Position, with arms bent and hands in front with one palm crossed and pressing against the other palm.

b. Move your hands high overhead, inhaling.

c. Exhaling, move your hands down slowly to your shoulders, then down slowly to your hips, resisting while moving both directions.

d. Repeat 8 times. Be sure to inhale as your hands move up and exhale as your hands move down.

e. Shake out.

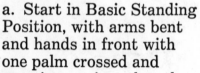

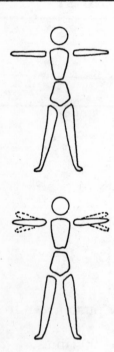

3. Arms/Chest I

a. Start in Basic Standing Position, with toes slightly turned out. Tuck your buttocks under and tighten your abdominal muscles.

b. Extend your arms out at shoulder level and, with palms down, move your arms forward in a circular motion.

c. Breathing rhythmically, start out with small circles and gradually make larger and larger circles as you count up to 10.

d. Release your arms to your sides when you have reached 10.

e. Extend your arms out at shoulder level and, with palms up, move your arms backward in a circular motion, gradually making larger and larger circles as you count up to 10.

f. Repeat 4 times forward and 4 times backward. Remember to breathe rhythmically and to keep your mouth slightly open.

g. Shake out.

4. Arms/Chest II

a. Start in Basic Standing Position, with toes turned out slightly. Bend your elbows at shoulder height, fingertips touching.

b. Exhaling, press your elbows back. Inhaling, return to the starting position and, exhaling, lead back with straight arms.
c. Repeat 10 times.
d. Shake out.

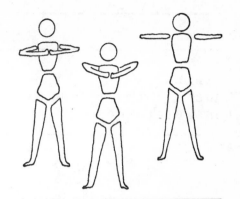

5. Upper Back

a. Start in Basic Standing Position, with feet straight forward. Clasp your hands behind your ears.
b. Flex your knees, round your back and, exhaling, bend forward with your elbows touching.

c. Inhaling, with your knees still flexed, slowly lift your shoulders and raise your elbows.
d. Return to the starting position.
e. Repeat 5 times, working up to 10 times. Remember to keep your buttocks and abdominal muscles tightly contracted.
f. Shake out.

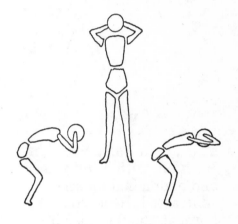

6. Walk or other cardiovascular exercise 8 to 10 minutes. Increase your pace slightly over the previous day's.

7. Basic Relaxation Exercise

a. Start in Basic Sitting Position, with knees bent.
b. Exhaling, slowly roll down to the floor, one vertebra at a time, until you are lying on the floor.

c. Let your spine come in contact with the floor, feet in line with your hips, arms outstretched, eyes closed. Rest until you feel relaxed.
d. Practice relaxation explained on page 100.

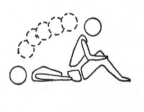

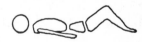

Warm up with 3 to 5 minutes of stretching from the first week's program.

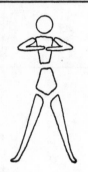 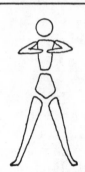 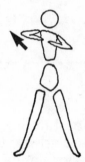

1. Waist Twist

a. Start in Basic Standing Position, with a tall spine and abdominal muscles contracted. Bend your elbows at shoulder height,

with fingertips touching. Inhale.
b. Exhaling, turn to your right, looking over your right shoulder and keeping your hips locked forward. Inhale.

c. Repeat the move, exhaling and turning to your left.
d. Repeat alternately 8 times on each side.
e. Shake out.

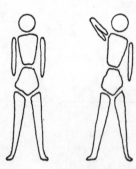 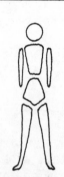 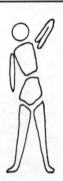

2. Waist Side Dips

a. Start in Basic Standing Position, with a tall spine, hips and abdominal muscles tucked under and thumbs touching the sides of your body.

b. Exhaling, draw your right thumb up the side of your body to your armpit, raising your elbow to the ceiling while letting the left arm slide down the side of your body.

c. Inhaling, draw your right thumb down you body to the starting position.
d. Repeat the move, drawing your left thumb up the side of your body.
e. Repeat alternately 8 times on each side.
f. Shake out.

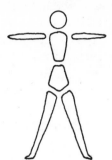 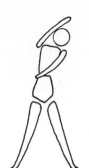 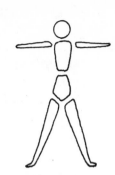 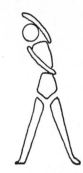

3. Waist Lateral Stretch I

a. Start in Basic Standing Position, with feet outside hip line and arms outstretched.

b. Exhaling, lower your right arm behind your back and bring your left arm up and over your head to the right side, keeping the arm in line with your ear and your palm down.
c. Inhaling, slowly return your arms to the starting position.

d. Repeat the move, raising your right arm to the left side.
e. Repeat alternately 5 times on each side.
f. Shake out.

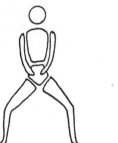 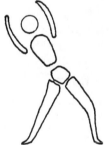 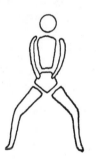 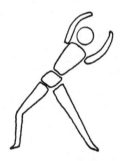

4. Waist Lateral Stretch II

a. Start in standing position, with feet outside your hip line, toes turned out, knees bent and hands in front of your body.

b. Exhaling, slowly move up and over to your right side, framing your face with your arms. Letting your weight shift to your left leg, straighten your right leg.
c. Inhaling, bring your arms back to the starting position in a wide circle, bending your knees and leading down with your

tailbone. Keep a tall spine and contracted abdominal muscles.
d. Repeat the move, moving to your left side.
e. Repeat alternately 5 times on each side.
f. Shake out.

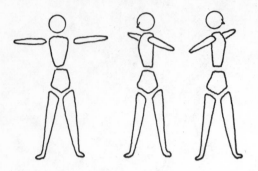

5. Waist Swing

a. Start in Basic Standing Position, with arms outstretched from shoulders and hips locked forward.

b. Breathing rhythmically, turn and look over your right shoulder and circle back, looking over your left shoulder. Remember to keep your hips locked forward.
c. Repeat 10 to 20 times.

6. Walk or other cardiovascular exercise 8 to 10 minutes, increasing your pace slightly over the previous day's.

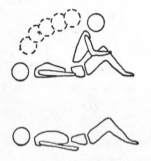

7. Basic Relaxation Exercise

a. Start in Basic Sitting Position, with knees bent.
b. Exhaling, slowly roll down to the floor, one vertebra at a time, until you are lying on the floor.

c. Let your spine come in contact with the floor, feet in line with your hips, arms outstretched, eyes closed. Rest until you feel relaxed.
d. Practice relaxation explained on page 100.

SECOND WEEK/DAY 4: ABDOMINALS AND LOWER BACK

The exercises that follow are designed to develop the abdominal area and your lower back. Remember that 85 to 90 percent of all lower back problems are due to weak abdominal muscles and poor posture.

Warm up with 3 to 5 minutes of stretching from the first week's program.

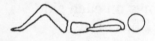 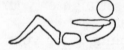 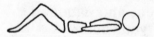

1. Upper Body Curl

a. Start in Basic Floor Position, with knees bent and arms at your sides. Contract your abdominal muscles and inhale.

b. Exhaling, tuck in chin and curl up, bringing your head and shoulders forward off the floor. Hold for 4 to 6 counts.

c. Inhaling, release and return to the floor.
d. Repeat 8 to 10 times. Be sure to contract your abdominal muscles.
e. Shake out.

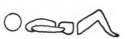 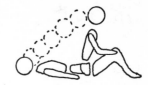

2. Bent Knee

a. Start in Basic Sitting Position, with knees bent. Inhale.
b. Exhaling, tuck in chin and roll down, starting at the base of your spine and curling down one vertebra at a time. Keep your chin tucked in throughout roll down.
c. Inhale. Exhaling, start curling back up, one vertebra at a time. Contract your abdominal muscles as you return to the starting position.
d. Repeat 8 to 10 times, working up to 20 times. If you are having difficulty curling up, place your hands on the floor, palms down, by your hips and push yourself up.
e. Shake out.

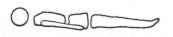 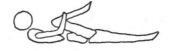 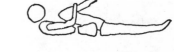

3. Lower Abdominal Muscles This exercise is almost identical to the abdominal exercise on page 120, except the head is raised in this one, making the exercise more difficult *and* more effective.

a. Start in Basic Floor Position, with legs extended and lower back pressed to the floor. Raise your head and shoulders. Inhale.
b. Exhaling, contract your abdominal muscles and draw your right knee to your chest. Inhale.
c. Exhaling, simultaneously extend your right leg and draw in your left knee.
d. Do 20 alternate moves. Be sure to keep your lower back pressed to the floor.
e. Shake out.

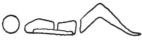 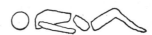

4. Reverse Torso Curl

a. Start in Basic Floor Position, with knees bent, feet flat on the floor and arms at sides. Inhale.
b. Exhaling, curl your hips off the floor, lifting one vertebra at a time until your lower back is off the floor.
c. Inhaling slowly, lower your hips back to the floor.
d. Repeat 8 to 10 times. This is an advanced move that will become easier as your abdominal muscles become stronger.
e. Shake out.

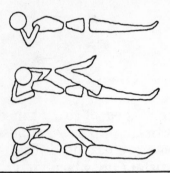

5. Elbow to Knee

a. Start in Basic Floor Position, with hands behind head. Inhale.
b. Exhaling, contract your abdominal muscles, then bring your left elbow up to meet your right knee.

c. Inhaling, return to the starting position.
d. Exhaling, contract your abdominal muscles, then bring your right elbow up to meet your left knee.
e. Repeat 20 times.
f. Shake out.

---

6. Walk or other cardiovascular exercise 8 to 10 minutes. Be sure to check your heart rate.

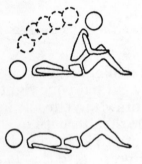

7. Basic Relaxation Exercise

a. Start in Basic Sitting Position, with knees bent.
b. Exhaling, slowly roll down to the floor, one vertebra at a time, until you are lying on the floor.

c. Let your spine come in contact with the floor, feet in line with your hips, arms outstretched, eyes closed. Rest until you feel relaxed.
d. Practice relaxation explained on page 100.

SECOND WEEK/DAY 5: HIPS AND BUTTOCKS

Warm up with 3 to 5 minutes of stretching from the first week's program.

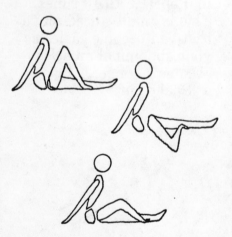

1. Bent-Knee Hip Rolls

a. Start in Basic Sitting Position, with left leg extended and right knee bent up with the right foot beside your left knee, your hands supporting out to side and back. Inhale.
b. Exhaling, roll your right knee out to the floor.

c. Inhale. Exhale as you bring your right knee over to the floor over your extended left leg.
d. Repeat this move smoothly 20 times on each side. If you have trouble getting your knee to the floor when crossing over, lift your hand into the air.
e. Shake out.

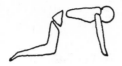 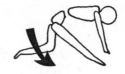

2. Leg Swings

a. Start in Basic Hands and Knees Position, with back level. Inhale.

b. With abdominal muscles contracted, exhale and extend your right leg out and forward to the right side.

c. Return your right leg to the starting position.
d. Repeat 10 to 15 times on each side.
e. Shake out.

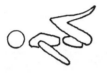 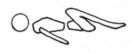

3. Hip Rolls on Back

a Start in Basic Floor Position, with arms outstretched at shoulder level, palms down. Draw your knees to your chest. Inhale.

b. Exhaling, roll your knees to the right side, letting your head roll to your left side and working to keep your left shoulder on the floor.

c. Inhaling, roll back to the starting position.
d. Repeat the move, rolling to the right side.
e. Repeat alternately 10 times on each side.
f. Shake out.

4. Hip Lift

a. Start in Basic Floor Position, with knees bent and feet flat on the floor. Inhale.
b. Exhaling, press your lower back into the floor, then to the count of 4, lift one vertebra at a time while raising your pelvis off the floor and letting your weight transfer to your shoulder blades. Inhale.

c. Exhaling, starting at the base of your neck, slowly return to the floor to the count of 4, lowering one vertebra at a time until your spine is in contact with the floor. Inhale.
d. Repeat 20 times, moving up to the count of 4 and returning down to the count of 4. Exhale as you lift; inhale, then exhale as you come down.

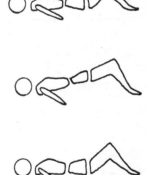

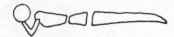 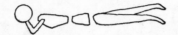 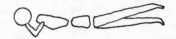

5. Leg Lifts

a. Start in Basic Stomach Position, with head turned to one side and hip bones in contact with the floor. Inhale.

b. Exhaling, contract your buttocks and the back of your right thigh, lifting your right leg with the energy in your heel.
c. Inhaling, return the leg to the floor.

d. Repeat the move on your left side.
e. Repeat alternately 10 times on each side.
f. Shake out.

---

6. Walk or other cardiovascular exercise 8 to 10 minutes, continuing to quicken your pace.

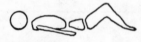

7. Basic Relaxation Exercise

a. Start in Basic Sitting Position, with knees bent.
b. Exhaling, slowly roll down to the floor, one vertebra at a time, until you are lying on the floor.

c. Let your spine come in contact with the floor, feet in line with your hips, arms outstretched, eyes closed. Rest until you feel relaxed.
d. Practice relaxation explained on page 100.

SECOND WEEK/DAY 6: INNER AND OUTER THIGHS

Warm up with 3 to 5 minutes of stretching from the first week's program.

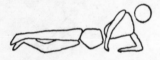 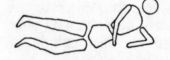 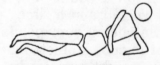

1. Side Leg Lift

a. Start in Basic Side Floor Position, with lower leg bent for balance. Inhale.

b. Exhaling, flex your top foot, keeping it parallel with the floor. Lift with the energy in your heel and go no higher than 45 degrees.

c. Inhaling, lower your leg back to the floor, keeping your foot flexed and your legs extended.
d. Repeat 10 to 15 times on each side.
e. Shake out.

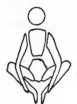 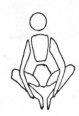

2. Adductor Stretch

a. Sit on the floor with your knees bent and the soles of your feet together. Position your elbows on the insides of your knees and your hands on your ankles. Inhale.

b. Exhaling, press your knees to the floor. Hold for 4 counts, breathing rhythmically and working against the resistance of the inner thighs. Inhale.

c. Exhaling, return your legs to the upright position against the resistance of your hands. Hold for 4 counts, breathing rhythmically, and inhale.

d. Repeat 10 times, 5 times up and 5 times down.

e. Shake out.

---

3. Inner Thigh Lift I

a. Start in Basic Side Floor Position, with top leg bent and your foot flat on the floor behind your extended leg. Flex the bottom foot and stretch the bottom leg. Inhale.

b. Exhaling, lift your bottom leg, keeping it extended and parallel with the floor.

Lift as high as is comfortable, but no higher than your bent knee. Inhale.

c. Exhaling, control and lower your leg to the floor. (Added resistance may be achieved by not returning your leg all the way to the floor.)

d. Repeat 10 times on each side.

e. Shake out.

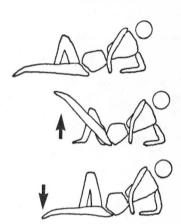

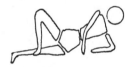 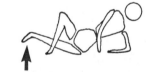 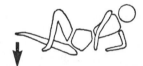

4. Inner Thigh Lift II

a. Start in Basic Side Floor Position, with top leg bent and your foot flat on the floor in front of your extended leg. Flex the bottom foot and stretch the bottom leg. Inhale.

b. Exhaling, lift your bottom leg, keeping it extended and parallel with the floor. Lift as high as is comfortable, but no higher than your bent knee. Inhale.

c. Exhaling, control and lower your leg to the floor. (Added resistance may be achieved by not returning your leg all the way to the floor.)

d. Repeat 10 times on each side.

e. Shake out.

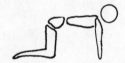 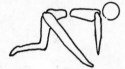 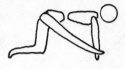 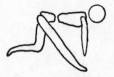

5. Kneeling Side Leg Lift

a. Start in Basic Hands and Knees Position. Contract your abdominal and buttocks muscles as you extend your right leg out to your right side. Inhale.
b. Exhaling, lift your leg. Hold for 4 counts, inhale and slowly lower to the floor.
c. Repeat 8 to 10 times on each side. Between sides, stretch back and release your muscles.
d. Shake out.

---

6. Walk or other cardiovascular exercise 8 to 10 minutes.

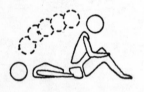

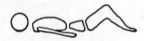

7. Basic Relaxation Exercise

a. Start in Basic Sitting Position, with knees bent.
b. Exhaling, slowly roll down to the floor, one vertebra at a time, until you are lying on the floor.
c. Let your spine come in contact with the floor, feet in line with your hips, arms outstretched, eyes closed. Rest until you feel relaxed.
d. Practice relaxation explained on page 100.

Warm up with 3 to 5 minutes of stretching from the first week's program.

1. Cross Over Leg-Toe Touch

a. Stand tall with your right leg crossed over your left, buttocks tucked under and abdominal muscles contracted. Inhale and reach over your head.
b. Exhaling, tuck in your chin and slowly lower your hands to your toes, bending your knees if necessary.

c. Flex your knees, contract your abdominal muscles, tuck your pelvis under and, inhaling, round up, one vertebra at a time.
d. Repeat 6 times with your right leg over your left leg and 6 times with your left leg over your right leg.
e. Shake out.

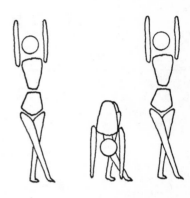

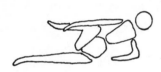 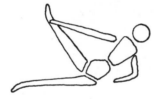 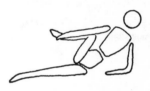

2. Leg Stretch

a. Lie down on your left side, supporting your body on your lower arm, lower leg extended and right knee bent up. Take hold of your right heel with your right palm, grasping from inside. Inhale.

b. Exhaling, straighten your leg as far as it will comfortably go while continuing to grasp your heel. Do not force this move.

c. Inhaling, bend your knee and repeat this move 4 times.
d. Now repeat the move 4 times on your left side.
e. Repeat alternately 4 "sets" on each side.
f. Shake out.

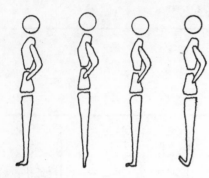

3. Toe Rise/Heel Lift

a. Start in Basic Standing Position, with pelvis tucked under, abdominal muscles contracted, hands on hips. Inhale.
b. Exhaling, rise up on your toes.
c. Inhaling, lower your heels to the floor.

d. Exhaling, rock back on your heels, keeping your body tall.
e. Inhaling, return your toes to the floor.
f. Repeat this cycle alternately 10 times on your toes and 10 times on your heels.
g. Shake out.

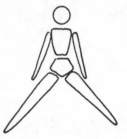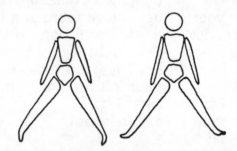

4. Ankle Circles

a. Start in Basic Sitting Position, with legs in a V position, supporting yourself with your hands beside you. Inhale.

b. Exhaling, contract your abdominal muscles and rotate your feet in toward each other. Inhale.

c. Exhaling, rotate your feet outward, pressing your little toes to the floor.
d. Repeat 10 times. Concentrate on making 180-degree arcs with your feet.
e. Shake out.

5. Leg Extender

a. Start in Basic Floor Position. Inhale.
b. Draw your left knee to your chest. Holding the back of your thigh, pulse 4 times in this bent knee position. Inhale.
c. Exhaling, extend your left leg upward, keeping your lower back on the floor. Pulse 4 times with your leg extended.
d. Return to the starting position.
e. Do this series 4 to 8 times with each leg.

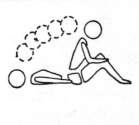

---

6. Walk or other cardiovascular exercise 8 to 10 minutes, increasing your pace over the previous day's.

---

7. Basic Relaxation Exercise

a. Start in Basic Sitting Position, with knees bent.
b. Exhaling, slowly roll down to the floor, one vertebra at a time, until you are lying on the floor.
c. Let your spine come in contact with the floor, feet in line with your hips, arms outstretched, eyes closed. Rest until you feel relaxed.
d. Practice relaxation explained on page 100.

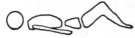

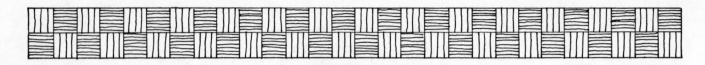

Pool Exercises

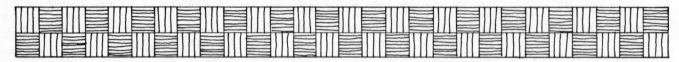

If you have access to a pool, there are many benefits that come from exercising in the water. The support of the water around your body—the floating feeling—decreases your body weight by 80 percent, allowing you to move more effortlessly and accomplish many exercises that would be difficult on land. On the other hand the resistance of the water forces you to intensify all your movements. And all the time the movement of the water around your body acts as a relaxing and beneficial massage; thus you are less likely to have sore muscles.

As on the ground, accompany your water exercises with your favorite music. But before getting in the pool, warm up with a few basic stretches from the first week of the *Fitness First* program. The following pool exercises are divided into three groups: upper body, waist and lower body. Select several exercises from each group each day. After completing each exercise, shake out and breathe in and out deeply a couple of times.

When exercising in the pool, swim some laps for your cardiovascular conditioning instead of walking. In addition to strengthening your heart, you'll be working your total body. Slow down by floating on your back awhile, gently stroking and kicking. Then finish with some relaxation exercises at poolside.

1a. Start in Basic Standing Position in shallow water with shoulders covered, arms outstretched to sides.
1b. Breathing regularly and keeping your abdomen contracted, make small forward circles with both arms. Repeat 10 times.
1c. Reverse this move, making small backward circles with both arms. Repeat 10 times.
1d. Shake out.

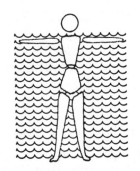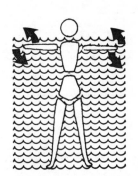

2a. Stand in shallow water with shoulders covered, knees bent and arms outstretched to sides. Inhale.
2b. Exhaling, press your arms down and, inhaling, pull them back up, keeping your upper body tall and contracting your abdominal muscles.
2c. Repeat 10 times.
2d. Shake out.

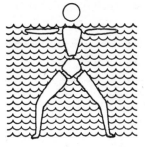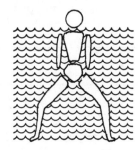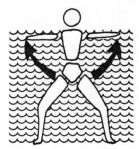

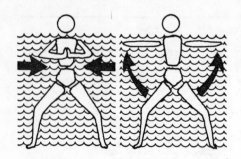

3a. Stand in shallow water with shoulders covered, knees bent and arms pressed together just below the water's surface, fingers together, thumbs up. Inhale.
3b. Exhaling, press your arms back, thumbs down, just below the water's surface, keeping your back tall and contracting your abdominal muscles.
3c. Inhaling, return to the starting position.
3d. Repeat 10 times.
3e. Shake out.

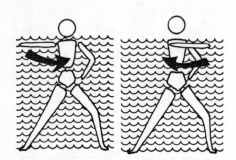

4a. Stand in shallow water with shoulders covered, left knee bent, right leg extended, right arm outstretched to the side with palm down and left hand on hip. Inhale.
4b. Exhaling, pull your right arm across in front of your body and up to the water's surface, keeping your abdominal muscles contracted.
4c. Inhaling, turn your palm down and pull your right arm back in front of your body, returning to the starting position.
4d. Repeat 10 times on each side.
4e. Shake out.

WAIST

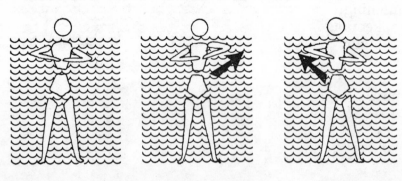

1a. Stand in shallow water with shoulders covered, elbows bent with fingers touching, hips forward, knees relaxed. Inhale.
1b. Exhaling, rotate your upper body to the right, looking over your right shoulder. Feel the energy in the tip of your right elbow. Inhale.
1c. Exhaling and keeping your elbows at shoulder height, follow through by turning to the left. Lead with the energy in the tip of your left elbow.
1d. Repeat 10 times.
1e. Shake out.

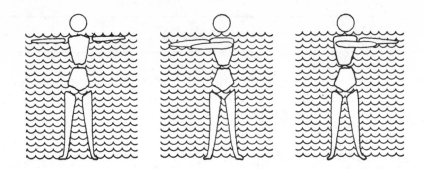

2a. Start in Basic Standing Position in shallow water with shoulders covered, arms outstretched and hands flexed up. Inhale.

2b. Exhaling, bring your left arm across the front of your body and stretch it out to the right side, reaching far enough to feel the stretch along your side.

2c. Inhaling, return to the starting position.
2d. Exhaling, repeat the move with your right arm.
2e. Repeat alternately 10 times on each side.
2f. Shake out.

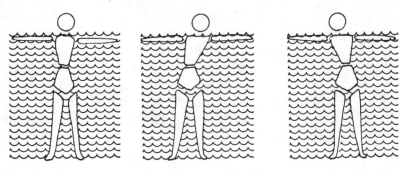

3a. Start in Basic Standing Position in shallow water with shoulders covered, arms outstretched to sides and your feet comfortably apart. Inhale.

3b. Exhaling, shift your upper body from side to side, leading with your fingertips and reaching as far as possible.

3c. Inhaling, return to the starting position.
3d. Reach alternately 10 times to each side.
3e. Shake out.

4a. Start in Basic Standing Position in shallow water with shoulders covered, arms down at sides and your feet comfortably apart. Inhale.
4b. Exhaling, slide your left thumb up the side of your body to your armpit as you let your right arm

go down your right side.
4c. Inhaling, return to the starting position.
4d. Repeat this move on the right side. As you relax on the exhale, feel the side stretch.
4e. Repeat alternately 10 times on each side.
4f. Shake out.

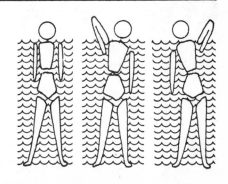

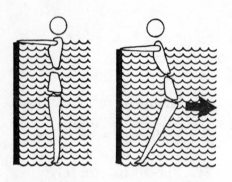

This move may be used between exercises to relax and release your body.

1a. Move to the side of the pool. Start in Basic Standing Position in shallow water with shoulders covered, holding onto the side of the pool with both hands, feet directly under your hips. Inhale.
1b. Exhaling, let your tailbone reach away from the side of the pool, arms outstretched. Feel your whole body stretch.
1c. Inhaling, return to the starting position.
1d. Repeat 6 to 8 times.
1e. Shake out.

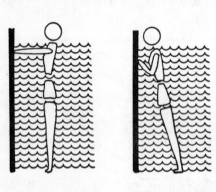

2a. Start in Basic Standing Position at the side of the pool in shallow water with shoulders covered, holding onto the side of the pool with both hands, feet directly under your hips. Inhale.
2b. Exhaling, slowly bend your elbows and lower your body to the side of the pool, keeping your body like a slant board from your shoulders to your heels.
2c. Inhaling, return to the starting position.
2d. Repeat 5 times, working up to 10 times or more.
2e. Shake out.

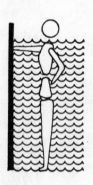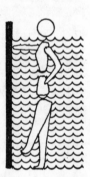

3a. Start in Basic Standing Position at the side of the pool in shallow water with shoulders covered, your right side toward the pool side and holding onto the side of the pool with your right hand.
3b. Contract your abdominal muscles and flex your left foot. Inhale.
3c. Exhaling, lift your left leg away from your right supportive leg, keeping your lifting in your heel.
3d. Inhaling, return to the starting position.
3e. Repeat 10 times on each side.
3f. Shake out.

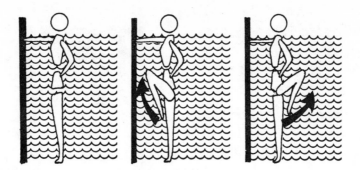

4a. Start in Basic Standing Position at the side of the pool in shallow water with shoulders covered, holding onto the side with your right hand and putting your left hand on your hip.

4b. Bend your left knee and put your left foot beside your right knee. Inhale.

4c. Exhaling, turn your left knee toward the side of the pool.

4d. Inhaling, turn your left knee away from the side of the pool, crossing it in front of your body.

4e. Repeat 10 times on each side.

4f. Shake out.

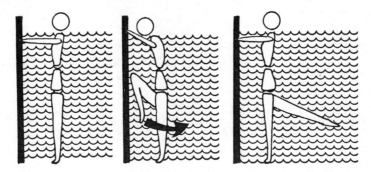

5a. Start in Basic Standing Position at the side of the pool in shallow water with shoulders covered, holding onto the side of the pool with both hands, feet directly under your hips.

5b. Tightening your buttocks, the backs of your thighs and your abdominal muscles, tuck your chin, round your back and draw your right knee to your chin. Inhale.

5c. Exhaling, lead back with the toes of your right foot until your leg is outstretched, lifting your head.

5d. Inhaling, swing your leg back slowly to the bent knee position, lowering your chin as you do.

5e. Repeat 5 times on each side, working up to 10 times or more on each side.

5f. Shake out.

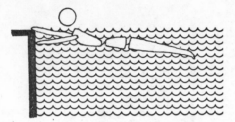 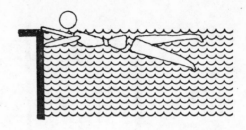

6a. Support your body horizontally at the side of the pool, with one hand in the gutter and the other on the side of the wall.

6b. Breathing rhythmically, contract your abdominal muscles and do a scissors kick back and forth.

6c. Repeat 10 times on each side.
6d. Shake out.

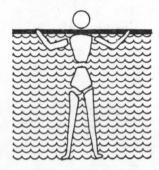 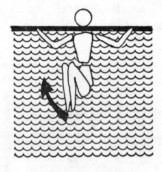 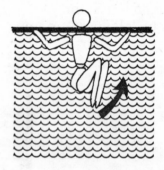

7a. Start in Basic Standing Position at the side of the pool, with your back to the side and holding onto the side with both hands.

7b. Breathing rhythmically, draw your knees to your chest, and roll to your right and then to your left, bringing your knees close to each elbow as you roll from side to side.

7c. Repeat 4 times on each side, working up to 10 times.
7d. Shake out.

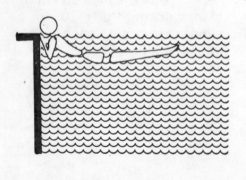 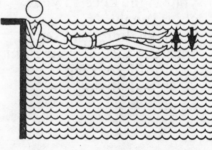

8a. Start in Basic Standing Position at the side of the pool, with your back to the side and holding onto the side with both hands. Slowly let your hips lift, contracting your abdominal muscles.
8b. Breathing rhythmically, flutter kick, starting the kick from your hips.
8c. Do about 20 kicks.
8d. Shake out.

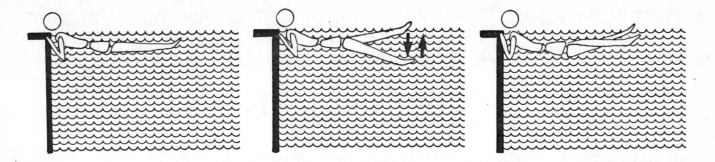

9a. Start in Basic Standing Position at the side of the pool, with your back to the side and holding onto the side with both hands. Slowly let your hips lift, contracting your abdominal muscles. Inhale.

9b. Exhaling and pushing against the water with the outsides of your feet, open your legs to a V position.
9c. Inhaling, return to the starting position by pressing against the water with the insides of your legs

and then crossing your right leg over your left leg, completing a scissors kick.
9d. Repeat this move, crossing your left leg over your right leg.
9e. Repeat 8 to 10 times.
9f. Shake out.

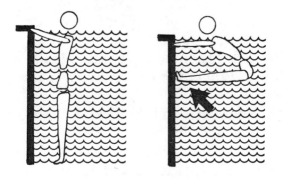

10a. Start in Basic Standing Position in shallow water with shoulders covered, holding onto the side of the pool with both hands, feet directly under your hips.

10b. Breathing rhythmically, slowly walk your feet up the side of the pool, feeling a total body stretch.

10c. Slowly walk back down.
10d. Repeat 5 times, working up to 10 times.
10e. Shake out.

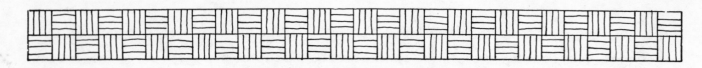

Bibliography

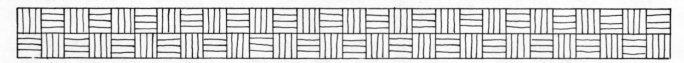

Church & Church. *Food Values of Portions Commonly Used.* 12th rev. ed. Philadelphia: J. B. Lippincott Company, 1975.

Jones, Jeanne. *The Calculating Cook.* Rev. ed. San Francisco: 101 Productions, 1978.

_____. *Diet for a Happy Heart.* San Francisco: 101 Productions, 1975.

_____. *Fabulous Fiber Cookbook.* Rev. ed. San Francisco: 101 Productions, 1979.

_____. *Secrets of Salt-Free Cooking.* San Francisco: 101 Productions, 1979.

U.S. Department of Agriculture. "Composition of Foods—Raw, Processed, Prepared." *Revised U.S.D.A. Agricultural Handbook,* No. 8, 1975.

U.S. Department of Agriculture. *Nutritive Value of American Foods in Common Units.* No. 456, 1975.

U.S. Department of Health, Education and Welfare. *Healthy People—The Surgeon General's Report on Health Promotion and Disease Prevention, Background Papers.* 1979.

U.S. Department of Health, Education and Welfare. "Disease Prevention and Health Promotion: Federal Programs and Prospects." *Report of the Departmental Task Force on Prevention, U.S. Department of Health, Education and Welfare.* September, 1978.

U.S. Senate Select Committee on Nutrition and Human Needs. *Dietary Goals for the United States.* 2d ed. December, 1977.

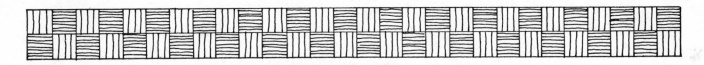

Index to Recipes

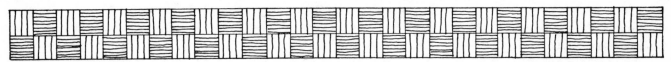

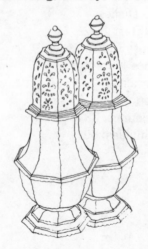

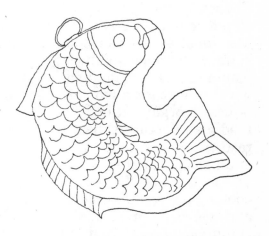

Jeanne Jones
Jeanne Jones is recognized as one of the leading writers, lecturers and consultants in the diet field. Her imaginative approach to entertaining, menu planning and food preparation and presentation has gained her an international reputation as a hostess. She created the menus and recipes in this book for the Canyon Ranch Vacation/ Fitness Resort in Tucson. Ms. Jones' first book, *The Calculating Cook*, published in 1972, was judged the best adult book of that year by the National Federation of Press Women. Her next book, *Diet for a Happy Heart*, was published in 1975, followed by *The Fabulous Fiber Cookbook* in 1977 and *Secrets of Salt-Free Cooking* in 1979. She is also the author of *Jeanne Jones' Party Planner and Entertaining Diary* and co-author, with Dr. J. T. Cooper, of the *Fabulous Fructose Recipe Book*. Ms. Jones serves as a consultant on recipe and menu planning and new product development for a number of health organizations, food manufacturers, health resorts and restaurants, and has appeared as a guest expert on diet and cooking on over 200 radio and television programs throughout the United States, Canada and Europe. She is an editorial associate of *Diabetes Forecast*, the official magazine of the American Diabetes Association, a member of the External Advisory Committee to the Diet Modification Program of the National Heart and Blood Vessel Research Demonstration Center in Houston and serves on the boards of directors of the San Diego County Heart Association and the Southern California Affiliate of the American Diabetes Association.

Karma Kientzler
As fitness director of the Canyon Ranch Fitness/Vacation Resort in Tucson, Karma Kientzler has developed an innovative program reflecting her upbeat philosophy that getting the body in shape and keeping fit is fun.
Karma Kientzler began her professional career in Bountiful, Utah, where she was AAU swim coach and eventually general manager and fitness director of the Community Swimming Pool.
In 1970, Karma went to California, where she developed, organized and coached the swim team for Poway High School in San Diego County and continued to train Red Cross instructors. Moving north to Ventura County three years later, she was introduced to a new approach to instruction wherein people are motivated to *enjoy* fitness. Incorporating this philosophy into her teaching techniques, Karma began creating unique exercise programs for all ages, beginning with "diaper gym."
By 1974, she and an associate had formed Fitness, Inc. and were instructing and coordinating workshops and fitness programs throughout the county. At this time they were asked to take over the fitness program for The Oaks at Ojai health resort. Six months later Ms. Kientzler was appointed general manager and assistant fitness director at The Oaks. Karma Kientzler moved to Tucson in 1978 to develop and direct the fitness program for the new Canyon Ranch Vacation/Fitness Resort.

Joe D'Addetta
A free-lance artist whose drawings appear frequently in *New Yorker* magazine, Joseph D'Addetta received his bachelor of arts degree from Jersey City State College and also studied at Parsons School of Design and New York University. He has worked as a graphic artist, a sportswear designer and an art teacher. His oils and watercolors have been exhibited in one-man and juried group exhibitions in the East. Presently he lives in San Francisco.